I0530462

The Manhattan Diaries Series

City-Slick Glamour
Manhattan's Makeup Guide
To Mesmerize

Manhattan Allure
Just Like That

The Manhattan Diaries Series

Manhattan Allure ~ Just Like That

1 – Unlock Manhattan: Master the Art of Lasting Impressions

2 – Behind the Velvet Rope: NYC's Grooming Secrets Revealed

3 – Skyline Secrets: How Manhattan's Elite Tame Their Tresses

4 – City-Slick Glamour: Manhattan's Makeup Guide to Mesmerize

5 – Urban Elixir: NYC's Proven Blueprint to Timeless Skin

Manhattan Vitality ~ Just Like That

6 – Eat Like an A-Lister: Manhattan's Ultimate Nutrition Guide

7 – Central Park's Fitness Hacks: How NYC's Best Shape Up

8 – Rise and Shine, Manhattan Style: Day-to-Day Luxuries You Can't Miss

9 – Soul of the City: Unlocking Serenity Amid NYC's Hustle

10 – New York Glow Up: Manhattan's Top Spa and Wellness Rituals

Manhattan Lifestyle ~ Just Like That

11 – Strut with Style: NYC's Guide to Unbeatable Fashion Confidence

12 – The Social Diary: How to Conquer Manhattan's Party Scene

13 – Manhattan Echoes: Reflecting Lifestyle from Living Spaces to Lanes

14 – Soiree Success: NYC's Ultimate Guide to Flawless Hosting

15 – New York Nurtures: Deepening Bonds in the City that Never Sleeps

16 – Romancing the Metropolis: Finding Love in NYC's Enchanting Streets

Manhattan Ambition ~ Just Like That

17 – Conquering the Concrete Jungle: NYC's Blueprint for Skyrocketing Careers

18 – Financially Fabulous: Manhattan's Secrets to Building Wealth with Style

19 – Hustle and Heart: NYC's Entrepreneurial Guide to Making It Big

20 – From New York City to the World: Jet Set Like Manhattan's Elite

21 – The Manhattan Magic: Discover the City's Indescribable Allure

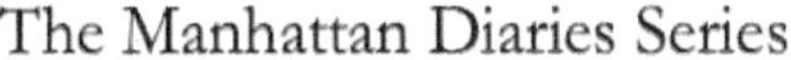

The Manhattan Diaries Series

City-Slick Glamour Manhattan's Makeup Guide To Mesmerize

Manhattan Allure
Just Like That

PAIGE MCCLINTE

Urban Chronicles Publishing House
an imprint of The Ridge Publishing Group
Coeur d'Alene, Idaho, U.S.A.

DISCLAIMER: The ideas, concepts, and opinions expressed in The Manhattan Diaries Series (hereinafter referred to as "Series") are intended to help readers make thoughtful and informed decisions about their lifestyle. This Series is sold with the understanding that author and publisher are not rendering medical advice of any kind, nor is this Series intended to replace the medical advice, nor to diagnose, prescribe, or treat any disease, condition, illness, or injury. It should not be used as a substitute for treatment by or the advice of a professional healthcare provider. It is recommended that before beginning any diet or exercise program, including any aspect of the Series, you receive full medical clearance from a licensed healthcare provider. Although the author and publisher have endeavored to ensure that the information provided in the Series is complete and accurate, the author and publisher claim no responsibility to any person or entity for any liability, loss, or damage caused or alleged to be caused directly or indirectly as a result of the use, application, or interpretation of the material in this Series, or any errors or omissions in the Series.

CREDIT: This book was written with limited assistance of ChatGPT, an AI language model developed by OpenAI. The collaboration provided unique insights and support in crafting content. The book cover was created using Midjourney tools and Adobe Photoshop, ensuring a visually captivating design.

Library of Congress Control Number: 2024919545

City-Slick Glamour: Manhattan's Makeup Guide to Mesmerize by Paige McClinte

ISBN: 978-1-956905-21-2 (e-book)
ISBN: 978-1-956905-20-5 (Softcover)

1. Health & Fitness / Beauty & Grooming. 2. Self-Help / Personal Growth / Success. 3. Self-Help / Motivational & Spiritual. 4. Lifestyle & Personal Style Guides. 5. Travel / United States / New York. I. Title. II. Series.

First Edition: September 2024

Printed in the United States of America

Contents

The Manhattan Diaries Series

DARE TO REIMAGINE YOURSELF . . .

21 Steps to Reinvent and Discover a Side of You Manhattan's Never Seen

The Manhattan Diaries Series presents:

Manhattan Allure—Just Like That mini-series (books 1–5)

Manhattan Vitality—Just Like That mini-series (books 6–10)

Manhattan Lifestyle—Just Like That mini-series (books 11–16)

Manhattan Ambition—Just Like That mini-series (books 17–21)

Meet the Author

https://www.LAMoeszinger.com

Meet the Publisher, Urban Chronicles Publishing House

https://www.NewYouniversityChronicles.com

Step into the whirlwind world of New York's glitzy underbelly, where the scintillating secrets and laugh-out-loud confessions of a metropolitan woman are laid bare by someone truly in the know. Through essays pulled from her chic "Manhattanite's Survival Guide—Success in the City," L invites us on an unforgettable strut from her glamorous youth, through her middle-aged mazes, and into her fabulous sixties.

For the juiciest tidbits about L's life, her "Manhattan Chronicles" blog is the place to be. This blog is an unfiltered dive into L's world, from her spiritual musings to her meticulous weigh-ins to her New Youniversity Chronicles—The Manhattan Diaries series—personal tales. Dive into her cosmos at her blog site: https://www.ManhattanChronicles.com.

The Manhattan Diaries Series

City-Slick Glamour
Manhattan's Makeup Guide To Mesmerize

Manhattan Allure
Just Like That

Introduction: Painting the Town Chic–Manhattan's Makeup Mastery Unleashed

Hello there, city dazzlers! When you step into the urban labyrinth of Manhattan, do you ever wonder how the elite achieve their mesmerizing makeup looks? Do you strut through the city streets with the confidence of a true New Yorker, or are you still unraveling the secrets to Manhattan's makeup mastery? Well, dear readers, the city holds a treasure trove of makeup secrets, and I'm here to reveal them all in "City-Slick Glamour: Manhattan's Makeup Guide to Mesmerize."

In this captivating journey, I'm taking you behind the scenes of Manhattan's makeup mavens. Success in New York City isn't just about wit or navigating the concrete jungle—it's about creating a makeup look that turns heads at every chic event, from uptown soirees to downtown happenings. I've mingled with the upper echelons of society, attended exclusive gatherings, and unearthed the makeup secrets that keep Manhattan's finest looking their most alluring. But remember, true allure begins from within.

Consider this your invitation to a limited-edition of The Manhattan Diaries series, experience. Whether you savor this treasure trove over leisurely days, indulge in it week by week, or read it while sipping cocktails on Manhattan rooftops, the pace is entirely up to you. Picture yourself diving into a chapter with your morning latte or immersing yourself in the entire book during a weekend escape. Within these pages, you'll unlock the keys to becoming the master of your makeup destiny, and the mesmerizing allure that follows will leave you spellbound.

As we embark on this journey together, I'll be your confidante, revealing how effortlessly you can conquer the realm of Manhattan makeup. This guide isn't just about makeup tips; it's a rejuvenation of your spirit, your relationships, and your aspirations in the city. Join me in uncovering the secrets that will make your makeup look as enchanting as the city skyline. I'm not just dedicated to helping you master the art of Manhattan makeup; I'm here to ignite the confidence in your heart that propels you to your most captivating self. Embrace it, and the energy of New York will be yours to command!

My passion for this city-centric guide is born from my own personal journey, filled with highs and lows, passion and heartbreaks. Like many city dwellers, I had to blaze my own trail, sometimes veering off the well-trodden path. But today, I stand before you, ready to inspire you to conquer your city with your makeup as your armor, cocktail in hand.

As time sails on the Hudson River, our life paths inevitably intersect. For me, the whirlwind of career pursuits, downtown extravaganzas, and self-discovery converged with my love for the city, leading me to work with the Urban Chronicles Publishing House.

New York City's allure isn't limited to celebrities or trust fund beneficiaries; it's accessible to everyone, whether you're a chic twenty-something or a sophisticated sixty-something. Embrace this journey with me as we embark on a path to city stardom in this fourth step—The Manhattan Diaries series is a twenty-one step journey; twenty-one books to reinvent and discover a side of you Manhattan's never met.

"City-Slick Glamour" equips you with the tools to not only dream big but to seize those dreams. I'm here as your city guardian, ensuring you realize that everything you crave starts within. With this guide, enhance your soul with Manhattan's finest secrets, and watch as your dream job, penthouse, or perfect partner follows suit. If you've got city-sized dreams, this series is your key to unlocking them! I've witnessed friends rise to stardom time and time again, proving that as you align within, the city will reflect it back in glitz and glamour. That's a promise straight from the heart of New York.

Relying on The Manhattan Diaries series has always been my lifeline. Whenever the city threw a curveball my way, this series steered me right back to my radiant path. The allure of always being on top keeps me coming back to these pages, and trust me, it's far more exhilarating than settling for mediocrity.

With every page you turn, you'll discover the blueprint, insider secrets, and the support you need to make your journey an exhilarating adventure. This series is tailored for everyone, from those seeking a fabulous career to social butterflies and empire builders.

There are countless ways to rise in the Big Apple, but if you're looking for the chicest route, it's right here in The Manhattan Diaries. Immerse yourself in its treasures while reciting positive mantras, and let the city's vibrancy chase away any doubts; and, in this case, allowing your makeup to become your ultimate statement piece. To truly reign, sometimes we need to shed our old makeup routines and embrace our most radiant selves.

Navigating the City with The Manhattan Diaries

Welcome to "City-Slick Glamour: Manhattan's Makeup Guide to Mesmerize." Think of this edition of The Manhattan Diaries as your personal cosmopolitan diary, as interactive as an invitation to Manhattan's most exclusive soirees. Each chapter is enriched with journal pages, waiting for your Manhattan musings and anecdotes. Whether you want to record the day's chic highlights in your "Beauty Chronicles" or delve into deep reflections in your "Beauty Confessions," these pages are yours to fill—see Cocktails and Chronicles: "Journal Pages: Pen Your Tales."

But . . .

1. Before you start penning your thoughts, take a moment to breathe. Close your eyes and, in that quiet moment, express a heartfelt "thank you" to the city that never sleeps. Feel that rush of gratitude, as if you've just been given a front-row seat to New York Fashion Week. Let that "thank

you" resonate deep within your heart—because that, my dear readers, is the magic of Manhattan.

2 Begin by detailing the fabulous strides you've made since delving into the last glamorous advice you've received. Write them down under "Completed Tasks," and relish in the feeling of owning every room you walk into with your captivating makeup.

3 Once you've celebrated your beauty triumphs, turn the page to "Action Items" and outline your aspirations. Reflect on what's left to conquer in your beauty journey, capturing your next steps in this transformational saga.

Throughout The Manhattan Diaries series, you'll encounter timeless "inspirational quotes" that are as iconic as Manhattan's skyline. These pearls of wisdom are your city mantras. Savor them, recite each word as if you're toasting at an Upper East Side salon, and let them resonate deep within your urban soul.

As you approach the end of each guide, you'll discover a "City Roundup." Here, you'll find a chic recap summarizing all the insider tips from your city escapade, ensuring you never miss a New York beauty minute.

So, get ready to unlock the secrets of Manhattan's beauty elite, darlings. Behind the cityscape lies a world of glamour, style, and endless possibilities. It's time to let your beauty shine as brightly as the city lights.

City-Slick Glamour: Manhattan's Makeup Guide to Mesmerize

Indulge in the captivating allure of Manhattan's high-society glamour with "City-Slick Glamour: Manhattan's Makeup Guide to Mesmerize," the fourth installment in The Manhattan Diaries series. If you're on the quest for an extraordinary life, dear readers, consider this your next essential step.

In "City-Slick Glamour," you'll unveil the secrets to achieving that upscale, polished look that sets you apart in the bustling heart of the city. Imagine a face that radiates wealth and sophistication, where not a hint of greasiness or mask-like artificiality can be found. This guide is your gateway to flawless makeup and foundation application, promising a photo finish look that will leave everyone mesmerized.

Join me on this enchanting journey where we'll explore the art of city-slick glamour. With the insights and techniques revealed within these pages, you'll master the art of makeup, ensuring that every day is your red carpet moment. So, let "City-Slick Glamour: Manhattan's Makeup Guide to Mesmerize" be your guide to achieving that captivating, flawless appearance that befits the elite of Manhattan. Your extraordinary life awaits!

Meet the Maestros Behind the Curtain

Welcome to the glittering realm of The Manhattan Diaries series, penned by an eclectic group of scribes who know how to make words shimmer just like that Midtown skyline. Each of these writers possesses the kind of Manhattan moxie that's as electrifying as a Saturday night at Studio 54. Picture the literary equivalent of the fabulous foursome from "Sex and the City," but with a little extra Manhattan mascara.

Our authors, darlings, aren't just writers; they're connoisseurs of all things NYC, dishing out stories with the precision of a Fifth Avenue stylist crafting the perfect blowout. Their tales are imbued with the kind of insider knowledge only those who've sipped martinis at the city's most secretive spots can truly understand.

So, as you delve into the pages of The Manhattan Diaries know that you're not just reading words, you're sipping on the prose of New York's finest literary mixologists. Here's to a journey as sparkling and unforgettable as a New York night out. Cheers, darling!

Behind the Scenes with the Urban Chronicles Publishing House

In the whirlwind of New York's high society, the Urban Chronicles Publishing House has emerged as the ultimate style sage for modern-day self-help. Over a cosmopolitan-fueled decade, they've become the city's go-to curators for crafting that sought-after, enviable life. The Manhattan Diaries? Envision it as your exclusive, VIP backstage pass, dripping with Upper East Side allure.

If you've ever pictured yourself sashaying through Manhattan with poise, if you've craved that skyline backdrop to your impeccable life, or if you simply seek the secrets whispered in the plush corners of the city's most exclusive clubs—The Manhattan Diaries is your ticket. Crafted under the elite banner, Urban Chronicles Publishing House, this imprint doesn't just offer you insights; it's your personal invite to the city's most glamorous circles.

- **Forever en Vogue**. Everyone, from the Wall Street moguls to the aspiring Broadway stars, dreams of basking in New York's radiant glow, of living a life drenched in style and substance. The wisdom in The Manhattan Diaries is as timeless as a Fifth Avenue romance, ensuring you're always en vogue.
- **A Blueprint for the Elite**. Nestled within these pages are the golden rules of city living, from mastering the cocktail chatter to undergoing a dazzling reinvention. Whether you're a seasoned socialite, an ambitious parent, or a fresh-eyed dreamer, these guides have something to make your heart race a little faster.
- **The Perfect Accessory**. Their petite stature makes these guides a seamless fit for your Prada clutch or your gym tote. Think of them as your urban survival kit—a blend of wisdom and wit that's as crucial as your red lipstick for those Manhattan nights.

Take a sip of this rich concoction, and let the Urban Chronicles Publishing House unlock Manhattan, unveiling a New York you only dreamed of. Welcome to the allure of the elite, darling.

Unveiling The Ridge Publishing Group

Picture The Ridge Publishing Group as the rising star on New York's literary and entertainment horizon. Envision an eclectic empire—books, cinema, and board games—setting the stage to become the world's haute couture of theological discourse. Think Fifth Avenue for theological resources: luxurious, elite, and unparalleled.

Dive into their esteemed collections. They hold the keys to the illustrious Guardians of Biblical Truth Publishing Group and the evocative New Narrated Study Bible (NNSB) series. Delve deeper and find the Hoyle Theology Publishing Group and its opulent Hoyle Theology Encyclopedia—a treasure trove for the cerebral sophisticate. And for those who like their theology paired with a cinematic flair, there's the Documentaries in Print Publishing Group with its tantalizing series like Defending the Faith. And, of course, for those cocktail nights with a side of divine strategy, the Heaven's Seminary board games and card decks offer a chic twist.

But that's not all. The Ridge Publishing Group is more than a theological publishing powerhouse; it's a brand. Alongside its flagship, it flaunts trendy imprints: AuthorsDoor Group and the AuthorsDoor Leadership program (check them out at the glamorous digital boulevard of https://www.AuthorsDoor.com), the ritzy Urban Chronicles Publishing House and New Youniversity Chronicles (make your reservation at https://www.NewYouniversityChronicles.com), and the novel delights of Ethan Fox Books (sip your martini and browse https://www.EthanFox Books.com).

For a sneak peek into the world where theology meets Manhattan glamour, rendezvous at their digital penthouse: https://www.RidgePublishingGroup.com. It's theology made chic.

A NOTE TO THE READER

Typos in this book? Errors (and inconsistencies) can get through proofreaders, so if you do find any typos or grammatical errors in this book, I'd be very grateful if you could let me know using this email address typos@LAMoeszinger.com. Thank you ☺

Bright Lights, Big City, Bold Brows: Perfecting the Frame of Your Face

Manhattan, a city that doesn't just revel in its grandeur—it flaunts it, with each boulevard echoing tales of dreams, dramas, and the deliciously daring. In this theater of life, it's not only about playing your part; it's about owning it—with panache, precision, and that perfect arch of the brow.

Visualize this: As you sashay down the iconic Fifth Avenue, it's not just the shimmer of your jewels or the cut of your attire that captivates. It's the bold statement made by your brows, framing your face like the marquee of a Broadway show. That, darling, is the Manhattan Gaze of Distinction, a declaration of self-assured beauty, unapologetic and unforgettable.

In this tantalizing chapter of The Manhattan Diaries, we delve deep into the world of brow artistry. From the natural, feathery strokes gracing the boho souls of Greenwich Village to the meticulously sculpted arches fitting the mavens of Madison Avenue, you'll unearth the craft of creating the perfect brow statement.

Yet, this journey isn't merely skin-deep. It's about capturing Manhattan's essence, about reflecting its myriad moods—its high-fashion highs and its reflective, introspective moments. It's about understanding that while skyscrapers define the city's silhouette, it's the brows that frame its face.

Accompany me, as we navigate the studios of Manhattan's brow virtuosos, feeling the passion, the precision, the art and the architecture of every brush and tweeze. Because in Manhattan, every glance, every expression, every subtle lift of the brow is a narrative waiting to be unveiled. Welcome to The Manhattan Diaries—where your brows can be as iconic as the twinkling city lights.

The Manhattan Gaze of Distinction

In the heart of New York City, where dreams are as high as the towering skyscrapers and the streets pulse with an unyielding energy, there lies a subtle yet powerful expression of style and confidence—The Manhattan Gaze of Distinction. It's not just a look; it's an attitude, a statement made with the bold arches of perfectly sculpted brows. Here, in the city that never sleeps, your brows are not just a feature; they are the marquee of your personal Broadway show.

- **The High Fashion Arch: Uptown Elegance**. In the polished corridors of Upper Manhattan, the brows speak of sophistication and high fashion. Meticulously sculpted, they are a tribute to the city's haute couture, as iconic as the designer labels that grace Fifth Avenue.

- **The Bohemian Stroke: Downtown Vibes**. Down in the eclectic streets of Greenwich Village, the brows take on a more natural, feathery form. Here, they tell stories of artistic souls and bohemian spirits, echoing the free-spirited energy of downtown.

- **The Power Brow: Corporate Chic.** In the financial heart of the city, brows are bold and empowering. They mirror the towering skyscrapers of Wall Street, representing strength, determination, and the unyielding ambition of Manhattan's corporate warriors.

- **The Trendsetter's Curve: Fashion Forward**. In the trendsetting locales of SoHo and the East Village, brows become the forefront of avant-garde beauty. Edgy, innovative, and daringly different, they reflect the cutting-edge styles and vibrant youth culture of these neighborhoods.

- **The Vintage Flair: Retro Glam**. In the nostalgic corners of Manhattan's vintage scenes, brows hark back to the golden eras of glamour. Inspired by the timeless beauty of classic Hollywood, these brows are all about bringing the elegance of the past into the present, with a touch of modern sass.

- **The Minimalist Approach: Sleek and Simple**. In the minimalist enclaves of the city, where less is more, the brows are kept sleek and unassuming. They speak to a refined aesthetic, where the beauty lies in simplicity and understated elegance, echoing the clean lines of modern architecture.
- **The Artistic Twist: Gallery Chic**. Among the city's art districts, brows become a medium of self-expression akin to the masterpieces adorning gallery walls. Here, they are not just groomed but creatively enhanced, embodying the innovative spirit of Manhattan's vibrant art scene.
- **The Celebrity Inspired: Star-Studded Styles**. In the celebrity-frequented hotspots, brows are influenced by the glamour and glitz of the entertainment world. These brows are bold and beautiful, often setting trends and defining what's next in the realm of high-profile beauty.
- **The Multicultural Mix: Melting Pot Magic**. Reflecting Manhattan's diverse cultural tapestry, these brows blend various global beauty standards to reflect the city's vibrant multiculturalism.

In Manhattan, every brow is a canvas, reflecting the rich tapestry of the city's soul. These brows are more than just a beauty statement; they are a celebration of individuality and the essence of Manhattan itself. From the polished arches of uptown to the carefree strokes of downtown, each style is a chapter in the ongoing story of this magnificent city. In the Manhattan Gaze of Distinction, every furrow, lift, and arch is a testament to the city's indomitable spirit—bold, unapologetic, and forever captivating.

Completed Tasks: Gaze of Distinction Activities

Inspirational Quote

THERE IS NOTHING STRONGER IN THE WORLD THAN GENTLENESS. — Han Suyin

Action Items: Intentions and Thoughts

Brow Artistry Across Boroughs

In the sprawling expanse of New York City, where each borough boasts its own rhythm and soul, there exists a fascinating mosaic of style and self-expression—Brow Artistry. This is not just about grooming; it's a celebration of identity, a vivid illustration of the city's diverse character, painted through the subtle art of brow styling. From the chic streets of Manhattan to the eclectic corners of Brooklyn, each borough tells its own story, not just through its streets and skyline, but through the arches and contours of its residents' brows.

- **Manhattan's Metropolitan Chic: The High-Fashion Arch**. In the fast-paced lanes of Manhattan, brows are as much a fashion statement as the designer outfits gracing Fifth Avenue. Precise, polished, and unapologetically bold, they reflect the city's flair for high fashion and the unceasing ambition of its inhabitants.
- **Brooklyn's Bohemian Brush: The Artistic Feather**. Brooklyn, with its laid-back vibe and artistic heartbeat, sports brows that are as unique and varied as its street art. Soft, feathery, and effortlessly cool, they echo the borough's spirit of individuality and creative freedom.
- **Queen's Cultural Tapestry: The Multicultural Meld**. In the culturally rich borough of Queen's brows become a canvas for global beauty standards. Here, the artistry is diverse and dynamic, reflecting the myriad of cultures and ethnicities that make Queens a melting pot of international charm.
- **The Bronx's Bold Statement: The Unconventional Bold**. In the Bronx, where raw energy meets urban grit, the brows are as bold and resilient as the borough itself. Unconventional and striking, they speak to the strength and fearless spirit of its people.

- **Staten Island's Subtle Elegance: The Understated Curve**. The brows of Staten Island tell a tale of understated elegance. Less about making a statement and more about enhancing natural beauty, they reflect the borough's quieter, more laid-back approach to city life.
- **Harlem's Heritage Highlight: The Classic Sweep**. Harlem, renowned for its rich history and vibrant arts scene, showcases brows that are both classic and expressive. These brows carry a sweep of elegance that mirrors the neighborhood's jazz-infused nights and its storied streets of historical significance.
- **Greenwich Village's Trendsetting Twist: The Modern Minimalist**. In the heart of Greenwich Village, where modernity meets rich history, brows are minimalistic yet trendy, reflecting the area's reputation as a hub for forward-thinking artists and intellectuals. Subtle yet impactful, these brows mirror the innovative and trendsetting spirit of its residents.
- **Financial District's Precision Lines: The Tailored Trim**. In the Financial District, brows are meticulously shaped, reflecting Wall Street's polished professionalism with sharp, clean lines that exude confidence.

In New York City, every brow, like every street, has a story to tell. These varied styles of brow artistry across boroughs are not just about beauty trends; they are a reflection of the diverse tapestry of life that makes this city a kaleidoscope of cultures, personalities, and stories. From the polished arches of Manhattan to the bohemian strokes of Brooklyn, each brow is a testament to the individuality and collective spirit of New York. In this city of endless possibilities, the way one styles their brows is more than a personal choice; it's a declaration of who they are, where they belong, and the unique narrative they contribute to the ever-evolving saga of New York City.

Completed Tasks: Brow Artistry Activities

Inspirational Quote

THOUGHT IS THE WIND, KNOWLEDGE THE SAIL, AND MANKIND THE VESSEL. — Augustus Hare

Action Items: Intentions and Thoughts

More Than Skin Deep

In the dazzling array of New York City's beauty and fashion scene, there's a story that goes far beyond the surface—a tale spun not just from the threads of fabric but from the very arches of our brows. This narrative isn't just skin deep; it's an intimate journey through self-expression, where each brow is a subtle yet profound reflection of the city's multifaceted soul. In the grand theater of Manhattan, where every street corner is a stage and every face in the crowd a character, the art of brow styling becomes a way of weaving personal stories into the city's vibrant tapestry.

- **The Expression of Identity: A Mark of Individuality**. In the myriad expressions of New York's inhabitants, brows stand as a bold declaration of individuality. Whether sharp and defined or soft and natural, they are a form of self-expression, as unique and varied as the personalities they accentuate.
- **The Language of Mood: The Emotional Palette**. Brows do more than frame the eyes; they speak the language of emotion. A subtle furrow can convey deep thought, a gentle arch a sense of wonder. In this city of unspoken narratives, brows are the silent communicators of our innermost feelings and moods.
- **The Reflection of Eras: A Journey Through Time**. As we stroll through the streets of New York, the brows we see are not just contemporary choices; they are echoes of times past. From the thin, penciled lines of the roaring '20s to the bold, bushy styles of the '80s, brows are a reflection of the fashion and cultural shifts that have shaped the city.
- **The Symbol of Trends: The Pulse of Fashion**. The evolution of brow styles in Manhattan is a testament to the ever-changing trends of the fashion world. Each curve and contour reflects the city's pulse, its constant movement at the forefront of style and beauty.

- **The Art of Precision: Craftsmanship and Care**. Behind every perfectly styled brow is a story of craftsmanship and care. It's an art form, where precision and attention to detail speak to the dedication and skill of those who shape them, just as architects shape the city's skyline.
- **The Canvas of Diversity: A Cultural Mosaic**. In NYC, each eyebrow style represents a snippet of the city's rich cultural mosaic. Thick, thin, feathered, or drawn, each style carries cultural significance and diversity, mirroring the city's global influences and the myriad backgrounds of its people.
- **The Expression of Rebellion: Symbols of Change**. Brows often act as symbols of rebellion and societal change. From punk-inspired stark shapes to the minimalist trends sparked by counter-cultural movements, brows in NYC often reflect the city's revolutionary spirit and its history of challenging norms.
- **The Gateway to Connection: Bridging Communities**. Beyond aesthetics, brow artistry in NYC facilitates connections, serving as a common thread among diverse communities. They foster conversations and bridge cultural gaps, turning a simple element of beauty into a powerful tool for social unity and interaction.

In New York City, the story of brows is more than a tale of beauty; it's a narrative rich with emotion, history, and artistry. These arches do more than adorn the faces of those who walk the city's streets; they are the silent storytellers of identity, mood, and cultural evolution. In the kaleidoscope that is Manhattan, every brow—whether carefully plucked or naturally wild—is a brushstroke in the city's vast and vibrant canvas, a piece of the puzzle that makes New York not just a city of sights, but a city of soulful expressions.

Completed Tasks: More Than Skin Deep Activities

Inspirational Quote

AND WHEN I BREATHED, MY BREATH WAS LIGHTNING. — Black Elk

Action Items: Intentions and Thoughts

Behind the Scenes with Brow Virtuosos

In the vibrant heart of New York City, where every turn unveils a new spectacle, there exists a world seldom seen but immensely influential—the realm of brow virtuosos. These artisans, working in the shadows of the city's glittering lights, are the unsung heroes of beauty, the sculptors of those defining arches that frame the windows to our souls. Here, in their studios, a dance of precision and creativity unfolds, where each tweeze and brush stroke is a testament to their mastery and dedication to the art of brow styling.

- **The Alchemists of Arch: Masters of Shape and Symmetry**. In the hands of these brow artists, tweezers and brushes become instruments of transformation. They understand the delicate balance of shape and symmetry, crafting brows that not only complement facial features but also elevate them to new heights of elegance.
- **The Color Connoisseurs: The Palette of Perfection**. Beyond shaping, these virtuosos are adept in the art of color. Selecting the perfect shade to match hair and skin tone, they ensure that each brow is not just well-defined but also seamlessly integrated, enhancing the natural beauty of their clientele.
- **The Trend Translators: From Runway to Reality**. With a keen eye on the latest fashion trends, these brow experts translate high-fashion styles into wearable art. They bridge the gap between the avant-garde designs of the runway and the everyday looks of the city streets.
- **The Storytellers of Expression: Crafting Character and Charm**. Each brow they sculpt tells a story, a narrative of personality and style. These experts don't just shape brows; they craft characters, understanding that each arch and curve adds depth and expression to the face.

- **The Guardians of Health: Beyond Beauty to Wellness**. For these artisans, brow care is not just about aesthetics but also about health and wellness. They advocate for and practice safe, hygienic methods, ensuring that the beauty of their work is matched by the well-being of their clients.
- **The Innovators of Technique: Pioneering New Methods**. These brow virtuosos are not just followers of trends but pioneers in their field, constantly experimenting with new techniques and tools to refine their craft. Whether it's through microblading, threading, or tinting, they push the boundaries of what is possible in brow artistry.
- **The Educators of Elegance: Sharing Knowledge and Skills**. Beyond their service, these experts often take on the role of educators, sharing their deep knowledge of brow styling with aspiring artists and clients alike. Through workshops and training sessions, they spread the gospel of good brow maintenance, ensuring their legacy of precision and style continues to flourish.
- **The Curators of Confidence; Boosting Self-Esteem**. At the core of their work, these brow specialists understand that their craft does more than alter appearances—it boosts confidence. By customizing brows to match individual styles, these experts boost clients' confidence, enhancing both personal and professional lives.

Behind every perfectly styled brow in New York City is the invisible yet impactful touch of a brow virtuoso. These artists, working quietly yet passionately behind the scenes, are the true architects of the Manhattan Gaze of Distinction. Their studios are sanctuaries of creativity and precision, where each brow is a masterpiece in its own right. In the city that never sleeps, these brow maestros remain the unsung beacons of beauty, shaping not just brows but the very essence of style and grace in the bustling metropolis of New York.

Completed Tasks: Brow Secrets Activities

Inspirational Quote

LIFE WOULD BE INFINITELY HAPPIER IF WE COULD ONLY BE BORN AT THE AGE OF EIGHTY AND GRADUALLY APPROACH EIGHTEEN. — Mark Twain

Action Items: Intentions and Thoughts

Every Brow Tells a Story

In the ever-evolving tapestry of New York City, where each street corner buzzes with its own unique rhythm, there lies a subtle yet profound narrative—the story told by each and every brow. These arches are not mere adornments; they are the unsung narrators of personal histories, silent yet eloquent testimonies to the lives that unfold beneath the city's towering skyline. In Manhattan, where every gaze can tell a tale as captivating as any New York Times bestseller, each brow shape, each subtle life, is a chapter in the grand story of life in the Big Apple.

- **The Bold and Beautiful: The Tale of Confidence**. Bold, defined brows that don't just follow trends but set them, speak of a confidence that is quintessentially New York. They tell a story of ambition, resilience, and the unyielding determination to make a mark in the city that never sleeps.

- **The Natural and the Nuanced: The Whisper of Authenticity**. Soft, natural brows, gently enhanced, carry a narrative of authenticity and ease. These are the brows of those who stride through the city's parks and avenues with a comfortable sense of self, a quiet assurance in their own narrative.

- **The Sculpted and the Sophisticated: The Symphony of Style**. Precisely sculpted brows, arching gracefully, are like the high notes in a symphony of sophistication. They tell tales of elegance and refinement, of evenings at the Met and afternoons in galleries, a sophistication that is as much a part of New York as its skyline.

- **The Creative and the Colorful: The Canvas of Creativity**. Brows tinted in hues that defy convention speak of an artistic spirit, of a story painted in bold strokes of creativity and uniqueness. These are the brows of the East Village, of Brooklyn's creative hubs, where every color and shape tells a story of artistic daring.

- **The Fleeting and the Fashionable: The Rhythm of Trends.** Brows that change with the seasons, morphing with the latest trends, are the narrative of the city's fashion-forward, those who pulse to the rhythm of New York's ever-changing style scene.
- **The Refined and the Regal: The Elegance of Heritage.** Meticulously groomed brows that evoke a sense of history and tradition narrate tales of New York's rich cultural heritage. These brows reflect an elegance that ties back to the city's grand past, from historical landmarks to timeless Broadway shows.
- **The Bold and the Brave: The Mark of Pioneers.** Thick, unabashedly bold brows symbolize the pioneering spirit of those who shape the city's future. These are the brows of innovators and trailblazers, individuals who face the city's challenges with audacity and vision.
- **The Subtle and the Serene: The Whisper of the Understated.** Lightly touched, almost invisible brows speak of the unassuming yet assured individuals who thrive in the quiet corners of the city. Their stories are less about commanding attention and more about the peaceful, steady contribution to the city's rhythm.

In the city of a million stories, brows are the subtle yet striking narrators of the unsung tales of New York. From the bold strokes of confidence to the soft whispers of authenticity, every arch and angle tells a story, contributing to the rich, vibrant narrative of life in this city. They are the unwritten chronicles of New York, framing not just the faces but the very essence of the people who call this city home. In the grand narrative of New York, every brow, like every person, has its own story to tell, a unique thread in the beautiful, complex weave of this city's soul.

Completed Tasks: Brow Storytelling Activities

Inspirational Quote

FROM ITS BRILLIANCY EVERYTHING IS ILLUMINATED. — Guru Nanak

Action Items: Intentions and Thoughts

Action Items: Intentions and Thoughts

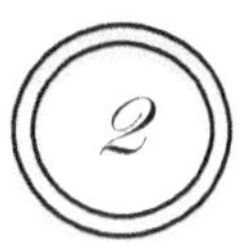

Metropolitan Mattes: The Secrets Behind an Oil-Free, Photo Finish Complexion

Manhattan, a city that doesn't merely live in the moment—it defines it, with each sunbeam and spotlight revealing tales of grit, glamour, and the golden rule: always be camera-ready. Here, where every reflection in a shop window could be your next profile picture, it's not about being flawless; it's about presenting your flawless self—with sophistication, savvy, and a skin game that's always on point.

Imagine this scenario: You're breezing down the legendary Fifth Avenue, and while your attire might be turning heads, it's the impeccable, matte finish of your skin that's truly stealing the show. That, darling, is the Manhattan Glow—subtle, sophisticated, and forever in vogue, a look that whispers elegance and screams confidence.

In this revealing chapter of The Manhattan Diaries, we'll pull back the curtain on the coveted secrets of the city's skin maestros. From the discreet rituals of the Upper East Side elite to the trendy hacks of downtown divas, you'll learn the art of achieving that perfect, photo finish complexion.

However, let's be clear: it's not solely about vanishing pores or keeping shine at bay. It's about echoing the city's own character—resilient yet refined, bustling but never chaotic. It's about navigating between the blinding billboards and serene park sunsets, understanding the delicate balance that is Manhattan's essence.

So, accompany me as we uncover the treasures tucked within the city's chicest salons and avant-garde ateliers. Dive deep into a world where skin care is not just routine but ritual. Because in Manhattan, every flash of the camera is a potential cover shot. Darling, it's time for your close-up in The Manhattan Diaries—where your complexion is as legendary as the city's skyline.

The Manhattan Glow Philosophy

In the mesmerizing landscape of New York City, where every street corner buzzes with a story, there exists a coveted secret whispered amongst the beauty mavens—the Manhattan Glow. It's a phenomenon that transcends mere skincare; it's an ethos, a way of life. This isn't just about having a radiant complexion; it's about embodying the sophistication and relentless energy of the city itself. The Manhattan Glow is the epitome of being camera-ready, not just in front of the lens but in every stride down the bustling avenues and serene park paths.

- **The Essence of Elegance: Subtle Sophistication**. At the core of the Manhattan Glow is the art of subtlety. It's not about glaring shine but a refined radiance that speaks volumes of one's grace and poise. This glow is a whisper of elegance, a quiet yet powerful presence that captures the essence of Manhattan's upscale charm.
- **The Science of Skincare: More than Skin Deep**. The philosophy behind this coveted glow is grounded in science. It's a meticulous blend of hydration, nourishment, and protection against the city's harsh elements. This approach is not just about surface beauty; it's about nurturing the skin from within, ensuring it reflects the city's vibrant health.
- **The Power of Presentation: Always Camera-Ready**. In Manhattan, the expectation to be perpetually photo-ready isn't just a trend, it's a lifestyle. The Manhattan Glow philosophy embraces this, ensuring that one's skin is always primed for the next impromptu photo op, be it on the streets, in the chic cafes, or atop the high-rise soirees.
- **The Art of Balance: Between Matte and Radiance**. Achieving the Manhattan Glow is about striking the perfect balance between a matte finish and a healthy sheen. It's understanding that true

radiance doesn't mean gloss, but a soft, luminous sheen that captures the city's dynamic light.

- **The Ritual of Self-Care: Luxury in Every Routine**. Central to the Manhattan Glow is the ritual of self-care. This involves indulging in luxurious skincare routines that are as much about pampering the spirit as they are about beautifying the skin. It's a daily homage to self-love, where each cleanse, mask, and moisturizer is a small yet significant celebration of oneself.
- **The Fusion of Nature and Technology: Harnessing the Best of Both Worlds**. This philosophy embraces the fusion of cutting-edge skincare technology with nature's finest ingredients. It's about leveraging scientific advancements for deep skin health while staying rooted in the natural world, creating a harmony that resonates with the city's blend of innovation and timelessness.
- **The Adaptability Factor: Skincare for Every Season**. The Manhattan Glow adapts with the changing seasons of the city. It involves tweaking skincare regimens to suit the sweltering summers and the biting winters, ensuring the skin remains radiant and resilient through snow, rain, and sunshine.

The Manhattan Glow is more than a beauty standard; it's a reflection of the city's heartbeat. It's about carrying the light of New York City on your skin—sophisticated, vibrant, and unapologetically alive. This philosophy goes beyond mere skincare routines; it's about embracing the city's energy, its relentless pace, and its undying spirit. In adopting the Manhattan Glow, one doesn't just wear the city's radiance; they become a part of its soul, a living embodiment of all that makes New York City an icon of style and elegance.

Completed Tasks: Manhattan Glow Activities

Inspirational Quote

IDEAS SHAPE THE COURSE OF HISTORY. — John Maynard Keynes

Action Items: Intentions and Thoughts

Secrets of the Upper East Side Elite

In the Upper East Side, an enclave where classic charm meets modern luxury, the secrets to flawless skin are passed down like cherished heirlooms. This is a world where beauty routines are more than mere maintenance; they're a ritual, a rite of passage, a testament to an exclusive legacy. The secrets of the Upper East Side elite aren't just about products or procedures; they're about a lifestyle, a dedication to preserving a standard of elegance and grace that has defined generations of Manhattan's finest.

- **Time-Honored Traditions: Legacy of Skincare**. Here, beauty secrets are family treasures, often passed from generation to generation. The focus is on timeless skincare rituals, with an emphasis on consistency and the use of tried-and-true ingredients known for their efficacy and gentleness.
- **The Luxury of Personalization: Bespoke Beauty Routines**. Customization is key for the Upper East Side elite. Skincare is deeply personal, with routines tailored to individual needs and preferences, often under the guidance of renowned dermatologists and estheticians who cater exclusively to this discerning clientele.
- **The Elixir of Youth: High-End Anti-Aging Solutions**. Anti-aging isn't just a concern; it's a craft. The elite invest in the most advanced treatments and technologies, from revolutionary serums to state-of-the-art non-invasive procedures, all to maintain their timeless, age-defying complexion.
- **Holistic Harmony: Beyond Skin Deep**. The Upper East Side's approach to skincare is holistic. It's not just about the external appearance but also about nurturing the body from within. This includes a balanced diet, regular exercise, and a focus on mental well-being, all contributing to the overall radiance of the skin.

- **Discreet but Decadent: Understated Elegance**. In this rarified world, less is more. The focus is on achieving a look that's effortlessly chic, never overdone. The mantra is clear: elegance is about being noticed without striving to be seen.
- **The Art of Subtlety: Refined Makeup Choices**. On the Upper East Side, makeup is an extension of skincare, used sparingly and strategically. The elite favor a "less is more" approach, opting for products that enhance natural beauty rather than mask it. Their makeup is as much about subtlety and refinement as their skincare, embodying an understated elegance.
- **Exclusive Sanctuaries: Private Spas and Salons**. The skincare sanctuaries of the Upper East side are as exclusive as they are exquisite. Access to private spas and members-only salons is a hallmark of this elite circle, where treatments are as luxurious as they are effective, offering a haven of tranquility and rejuvenation in the heart of the bustling city.
- **Preventive Philosophy: Proactive Skincare Regimen**. Prevention is a cornerstone of the Upper East Side skincare ethos. Rather than waiting to address issues as they arise, the elite focus on proactive measures—using sun protection religiously and embracing antioxidant-rich products—to maintain their youthful radiance.

In the hushed, luxurious corridors of the Upper East Side, beauty is a legacy, a whisper of the past echoing in the present. Here, the secrets to a perfect complexion are more than skin deep; they're a blend of tradition, innovation, and a holistic approach to well-being. The Upper East Side elite don't just maintain their beauty; they curate it, preserving the elegance and sophistication that define this illustrious corner of Manhattan. In this realm, every ritual, every product, every careful choice is a step in the timeless dance of grace and refinement—a dance as intricate and beautiful as the city itself.

Completed Tasks: Skin Deep Activities

Inspirational Quote

WHILE THERE'S LIFE, THERE'S HOPE. — Marcus Tullius Cicero

Action Items: Intentions and Thoughts

Downtown Divas' Trendy Hacks

In the pulsating heart of Downtown Manhattan, where the streets buzz with a rhythm all their own, the beauty ethos is as bold and eclectic as the divas who walk them. Here, the edgy enclaves from SoHo to the Lower East Side, skincare and beauty are not just routines; they are statements of individuality and rebellion. Downtown Divas, with their fingertips on the pulse of the latest trends, transform skincare and makeup into trendy hacks, making bold statements that are as daring as they are distinctive. In this world, beauty is not about conforming; it's about standing out.

- **The DIY Darlings: Innovative Home Solutions**. Creativity is king for Downtown Divas, who often turn to DIY beauty solutions. Homemade face masks, natural ingredient concoctions, and inventive skincare hacks are their arsenal, blending effectiveness with a personal touch.

- **Tech-Savvy Trendsetters: Gadgets and Gizmos Aplenty**. These divas are quick to embrace the latest in beauty technology. From advanced skincare tools to futuristic makeup applicators, they're always ahead of the curve, using technology not just for efficacy, but as a form of beauty expression.

- **The Bold and the Beautiful: Daring Makeup Choices**. For Downtown Divas, makeup is an art form. Bold colors, experimental looks, and unconventional techniques are their signatures. They don't shy away from making a statement, whether it's through a neon eyeshadow or a graphic eyeliner.

- **Sustainability Chic: Eco-Friendly Choices**. Conscious of their environmental impact, these trendsetters often opt for eco-friendly and sustainable beauty products. They prove that style and sustainability can coexist, championing brands and products that are as good for the earth as they are the skin.

- **Street Style Influencers: Fashion-Forward Skincare**. These divas know that true style starts with great skin. They are often the first to try out and popularize new skincare trends, from the latest in Korean beauty to the newest superfood-infused cream, always a step ahead in the skincare game.
- **The Revivalists: Retro Reimagined**. Downtown Divas have a knack for resurrecting and reimagining beauty trends from past decades. Whether it's a '90s-inspired grunge lip or a '70s disco eye, they blend retro charm with modern flair, proving that in beauty, everything old can be new again.
- **The Experimenters: Mixing and Matching**. These divas are not afraid to experiment. Mixing products to create custom blends, layering skincare in unconventional ways, or using makeup in multipurpose roles—their approach is all about personalization and discovering new ways to use traditional products.
- **The Wellness Warriors: Beauty From Within**. For these trendsetters, beauty is as much about inner health as outer appearance. Embracing wellness trends like yoga, meditation, and nutrition-focused diets, they ensure their beauty regimen is holistic, reflecting a glow that comes from within.

In the vibrant districts of Downtown Manhattan, the Divas' approach to beauty is a thrilling fusion of innovation, individuality, and audacity. They don't just follow trends; they set them. With each daring makeup choice and each creative skincare hack, they rewrite the rules of beauty, embodying the fearless spirit and avant-garde energy of downtown. In their world, every street is a runway, every sidewalk a stage, where beauty is not just seen but experienced, a dynamic expression of the bold, unapologetic essence of Downtown Manhattan.

Completed Tasks: Trendy Hacks Activities

Inspirational Quote

THERE ARE TWO WAYS OF SPREADING LIGHT: TO BE THE CANDLE OR THE MIRROR THAT REFLECTS IT. — Edith Wharton

Action Items: Intentions and Thoughts

Manhattan's Essence in Skincare

In the ever-changing, ever-moving city of Manhattan, where the skyline sparkles and the streets hum with a life all their own, the essence of the city is captured not just in its architecture and culture, but in the skincare rituals of its inhabitants. Manhattan's essence in skincare is a reflection of its character—resilient yet refined, bustling but poised. It's a dance between the high energy of city life and the serene, mindful practices that keep its people grounded. This is where skincare transcends the boundaries of routine, becoming a symbol of the city's spirit.

- **The High-Energy Hydration: Battling the Urban Elements**. The city's fast pace and environmental stressors call for skincare that protects and hydrates. Products rich in antioxidants and hydrating agents combat pollution and the hustle of city life, reflecting Manhattan's resilience in the face of constant movement.

- **The Serenity of Self-Care: An Oasis in the Chaos**. Amidst the city's rush, skincare routines become a moment of tranquility. Gentle, mindful practices like facial massages or aromatherapy-infused products embody the city's need for calm amidst the chaos, mirroring the peaceful sanctuaries found in its parks and quiet corners.

- **The Trendsetting Formulas: Innovation at Its Core**. Just as the city leads in fashion and art, it does in skincare too. Innovative, cutting-edge ingredients and formulations echo Manhattan's role as a trendsetter, constantly evolving and pushing the boundaries of beauty and wellness.

- **The Luxury of Timelessness: Classic Meets Contemporary**. In Manhattan, timeless beauty rituals merge with contemporary innovations. This blend of classic and modern approaches in skincare reflects the city's unique ability to honor its history while embracing the new and the now.

- **The Diversity of Skincare: A Melting Pot of Beauty**. Just like its population, Manhattan's skincare is diverse and inclusive. A range of products catering to different skin types, concerns, and cultural beauty practices mirrors the city's rich tapestry of people and traditions.
- **The Precision of Personalization: Tailored Skincare for Every Lifestyle**. In a city as diverse as Manhattan, one-size-fits-all is never the approach. Personalized skincare, tailored to individual lifestyles, routines, and skin needs, reflects the city's recognition of uniqueness and individuality. Whether it's for the bustling Wall Street broker or the creative artists in Greenwich Village, skincare in Manhattan is as personalize as the city's array of inhabitants.
- **The Fusion of Global Influences: Worldly Wisdom in Local Bottles**. Manhattan, a melting pot of cultures, brings the best of global beauty secrets to its skincare. From Asian beauty innovations to European skincare classics, the city's skincare embodies a fusion of worldwide beauty philosophies, mirroring its cosmopolitan and inclusive spirt.

Manhattan's essence in skincare is a dynamic blend of resilience, serenity, innovation, timelessness, and diversity—much like the city itself. It's a reflection of how the people of Manhattan live their lives, balancing the energy and excitement with moments of peace and self-care. In every jar, tube, or bottle, there's a piece of Manhattan's spirit, a testament to the city's ability to adapt, thrive, and lead in the ever-changing world of beauty and skincare. Here, skincare is more than just skin deep; it's a celebration of the city's heart and soul.

Completed Tasks: Mindful Practices Activities

Inspirational Quote

As we express our gratitude, we must never forget that the highest appreciation is not to utter words, but to live by them.
— John F. Kennedy

Action Items: Intentions and Thoughts

The Art of Skin Rituals

In the luminous glow of Manhattan's skyline, where every light tells a story, skincare transcends the mundane, becoming a revered ritual, a sacred symphony played out in bathrooms and boudoirs across the city. Here, in the metropolis of dreams and drama, skincare is not just a routine; it's an art, a daily performance where precision meets passion, and where every stroke, every dab, every gentle massage is a testament to self-love and city pride. In Manhattan, the art of skin rituals is a dance of elegance and efficiency, reflecting the city's blend of hustle and serenity.

- **The Morning Prelude: Awakening the Skin**. As the city stirs to life, the morning skincare ritual is like the first act of a ballet, gentle yet invigorating. Cleansing, toning, and hydrating with products that awaken and energize the skin, preparing it for the day ahead, mirror Manhattan's own awakening.
- **The Midday Intermezzo: Refresh and Protect**. Amidst the day's hustle, Manhattanites pause for a skincare intermission. A quick refresh with mists, the reapplication of sunscreen, or a dab of moisturizer—this midday ritual is all about protection and rejuvenation, echoing the city's dynamic energy.
- **The Evening Denouement; A Nighttime Indulgence**. As dusk falls over the city, the skincare routine becomes an indulgent denouement. Rich creams and serums, luxurious masks, and perhaps a facial massage, all work in unison to repair and rejuvenate the skin after a day in the city, much like Manhattan itself unwinds at night.
- **The Weekly Special: Deep Care and Repair**. Once a week, the skincare routine transforms into a special event. Exfoliating treatments, deep hydration masks, or perhaps a professional facial, offer a deeper level of care, reflecting Manhattan's penchant for weekly rituals, be it Sunday brunches or gallery openings.

- **The Holistic Approach: Skin and Soul in Sync**. In Manhattan, skincare is as much about the soul as it is about the skin. Incorporating elements of wellness, like meditation or yoga, into skincare routines, emphasizes the city's belief in the holistic connection between mind, body, and skin health.
- **The Seasonal Sonata: Harmonizing with the Seasons**. In Manhattan, skincare adapts to the changing seasons like a well-composed sonata. Lightweight, hydrating products for the sweltering summers and richer, more protective formulations for the harsh winters reflect the city's ability to harmonize with the rhythm of nature.
- **The Urban Detox: Cleansing the City's Imprint**. Recognizing the toll that urban living can take, Manhattanites incorporate detoxifying elements into their skincare. Purifying masks, pollution-fighting serums, and deep-cleansing routines act as a counterbalance to the city's frenetic energy, offering a skin detox that's as rejuvenating as a walk in Central Park.
- **The Expressive Finale: Personalization as a Signature**. In the art of skin rituals, personalization is key. Each individual tailors their routine to their skin's unique story and needs, much like how each New Yorker has their own distinct path and pace.

In the city that never sleeps, the art of skin rituals is a reflection of its heartbeat. Each cleanse, each application, each nourishing touch is a note in the melody of Manhattan life. It's a practice where elegance meets effectiveness, where the act of caring for one's skin becomes a celebration of self and city. In these rituals, Manhattanites find not just beauty but a moment of connection to themselves and to the vibrant city they call home. Here, skincare, is more than just maintenance; it's a love affair with the skin and the city, a daily ode to the beauty and rhythm of Manhattan.

Completed Tasks: Skincare Ritual Activities

Inspirational Quote

HEALTH IS THE GREATEST POSSESSION. CONTENTMENT IS THE GREATEST TREASURE. CONFIDENCE IS THE GREATEST FRIEND. NON-BEING IS THE GREATEST JOY. — Lao Tzu

Action Items: Intentions and Thoughts

Action Items: Intentions and Thoughts

Rooftop Rendezvous Reds: Lip Shades for Every Occasion from Day to Night

Manhattan, a city that doesn't just flirt—it seduces, with every sultry glance revealing tales of romance, intrigue, and the siren's call. Amidst this concrete jungle of dreams, it's not just about where you're going, but how you announce your arrival—with a swish of fabric, the right pair of heels, and the ultimate statement: a powerfully painted pout.

Picture this: You're dancing down Fifth Avenue, every corner a catwalk, every streetlight a spotlight. As onlookers are captivated, it isn't the flair of your ensemble alone that bewitches—it's the bold red that graces your lips. That, my dear, is the Manhattan Kiss, a declaration of audacity that speaks of passion, allure, and an invitation to the unexpected.

In this tantalizing chapter of The Manhattan Diaries, we'll dive into the world of reds, those beguiling shades that have ruled the hearts of Manhattanites from the art deco bars to the modern rooftop lounges. From the subtle hint of a daytime brunch berry to the brazen scarlet of a late-night liaison, you'll master the spectrum of reds that paint stories, desires, and ambitions.

But remember, this isn't just about hues—it's about attitude. It's capturing the pulse of Manhattan, swiping on the essence of moments, memories, moonlit nights, and sun-drenched days. It's painting both the romance of Central Park in autumn and the fervor of Broadway's brightest lights.

So, come along as we embark on a journey from the intimate corners of speakeasies to the glittering heights of skyscraper soirees, unraveling the secrets of the shades that can set hearts racing. Because, darling, in Manhattan, every smile, every word, every kiss is an event. Ready your lips for their standing ovation in The Manhattan Diaries—where your lip shade is as captivating as the city's nightscape.

The Daytime Flirt

In the soft, golden light of a Manhattan morning, when the city hums gently to life, there's a subtle yet undeniable allure in the air. It's the allure of the Daytime Flirt, a dance of elegance and sophistication played out on the sunlit streets. Here, amidst the clatter of coffee cups and the rustle of morning papers, the art of seduction begins with a whisper, not a shout. It's in this light that the right shade of lipstick—a muted yet mesmerizing red—becomes the silent herald of one's presence, a nod to the chic and playful energy of daytime in the city.

- **The Brunch Berry: Soft Hues for Morning Mimosas**. Imagine a leisurely brunch in the leafy enclaves of Central Park. The ideal red for this setting is a soft, berry hue, understated yet inviting, mirroring the freshness of the morning and the sweetness of the first sips of a mimosa.

- **The Business Chic: Polished Reds for Professional Poise**. For the power meetings and business lunches that pulse through the veins of Manhattan, choose a red that's polished and poised. A matte, muted red speaks volumes of professionalism, complementing the sharp lines of a tailored suit or a sleek pencil skirt.

- **The Casual Encounter: Flirty Tints for Daytime Dates**. On casual strolls through the bustling markets or quaint streets, a sheer red tint is the perfect companion. It's effortless, yet captivating—a flirtatious hint that pairs perfectly with the laid-back vibe of a sunny Manhattan afternoon.

- **The Art Aficionado: Cultured Shades for Gallery Hops**. For an afternoon wandering the galleries of Chelsea, opt for a sophisticated, deeper shade of red. It's a color that speaks of art and culture, as rich and complex as the canvases that adorn the white walls.

- **The Riverside Reverie: Subdued Reds for Waterfront Walks**. For a serene walk along the Hudson or East River, a subdued, coral-red shade is the perfect companion. It's a hue that reflects the tranquil blues of the water and the soft greens of the riverside parks, ideal for a peaceful yet stylish daytime outing.
- **The Urban Explorer: Vibrant Yet Approachable for City Adventures**. On days filled with urban exploration, from the historic streets of Lower Manhattan to the bustling avenues of Midtown, a bright but approachable red adds a pop of color. It's vibrant enough to stand out, yet subtle enough to blend with the day's energetic vibe.
- **The Cafe Chic: Elegant and Understated for Coffee Retreats**. For those moments spent in quaint cafes, reading or people-watching, a light, rosy-red with a hint of pink is the go-to. This shade is elegant and understated, perfect for enjoying a latte or a leisurely lunch, embodying the chic and relaxed atmosphere of Manhattan's favorite cafes.
- **The Morning Commute: Subtle Reds for the Early Rush**. As the city wakes and the rush hour begins, a subtle, almost nude red lipstick is the perfect choice. It's light enough to add a touch of grace as you navigate the bustling subways and streets. This hue complements the brisk pace and the emerging energy of a new day.

In the daytime dance of Manhattan, where every moment holds the promise of a new story, the right shade of red is your silent partner. It's a color that doesn't overpower but enhances, adding a touch of romance to the daily hustle. This Daytime Flirt is a celebration of the city's softer side, a playful yet elegant nod to the endless possibilities that unfurl under the gentle caress of the Manhattan sun. Here, in the daylight, every smile becomes a work of art, every glance a story, with just a hint of red.

Completed Tasks: Daytime Flirt Activities

Inspirational Quote

LET EVERY DAWN BE TO YOU AS THE BEGINNING OF LIFE, AND EVERY SETTING SUN BE TO YOU AS ITS CLOSE. — John Ruskin

Action Items: Intentions and Thoughts

The Evening Enchantress

As the sun dips below the horizon, Manhattan transforms into an enchanting playground of lights and shadows, where the evening brings its own brand of magic. It's in this twilight realm that the Evening Enchantress emerges, her presence announced not just by the swish of her gown but by the captivating allure of her lips. In the night's embrace, red lipstick is no mere adornment; it becomes a weapon of seduction, a bold statement of the night's intentions. From the intimate corners of dimly lit lounges to the pulsating heart of a rooftop party, the right shade of red is the enchantress's silent accomplice, weaving tales of intrigue and desire.

- **The Cocktail Hour Crimson: Bold and Sophisticated for Nighttime Soirees**. For the cocktail hours that sparkle with conversation and clinking glasses, a deep crimson shade sets the stage. It's bold, commanding attention, yet sophisticated enough to mingle with the refined elegance of Manhattan's elite lounges.
- **The Broadway Bold: Dramatic and Daring for Theatrical Nights**. On nights spent under the bright lights of Broadway, a vivid, daring red matches the drama of the stage. It's a color for the bold, for those who are not afraid to stand in the spotlight and embrace the theatricality of the city's vibrant arts scene.
- **The Rooftop Ruby: Glamorous and Radiant for Sky-High Affairs**. Atop the city's towering skyscrapers, where the night sky meets urban grandeur, a radiant ruby red is the choice du jour. Glamorous and captivating, it mirrors the sparkle of the city lights and the starry sky above.
- **The Late-Night Scarlet: Seductive and Bold for After-Hours Adventures**. In the late hours, as the city pulses with a more intimate energy, a deep scarlet shade becomes the confidant of the night owls.

This hue is seductive, perfect for those after-hours adventures that thrive in the city that never sleeps.

- **The Dinner Date Merlot: Intimate and Inviting for Romantic Evenings**. For those candlelit dinners at Manhattan's finest restaurants, a merlot red is the perfect companion. Rich and inviting, it adds an intimate touch to the evening, perfect for moments filled with soft music, fine wine, and whispered conversations.
- **The Jazz Club Burgundy: Sultry and Mysterious for Music-Filled Nights**. In the cozy, dimly-lit jazz clubs that dot the city, a burgundy shade sets the right tone. This sultry and mysterious hue resonates with the deep, soulful rhythms of the music, embodying the allure and mystique of a night spent swaying to the blues.
- **The Gala Garnet: Elegant and Dazzling for Formal Events**. For the grand galas and formal events that light up Manhattan's social calendar, a garnet red makes a dazzling statement. Elegant and refined, yet bold enough to stand out, it complements the luxurious gowns and sparkling jewels, making it the ideal choice for a night of opulence and celebration.

As night falls over Manhattan, the Evening Enchantress reigns supreme, her red lips a symbol of the night's endless possibilities. Each shade of red tells a different story—one of sophistication, drama, glamour, and seduction. It's more than just a color; it's a declaration of presence, a signifier of the enchantress's mood and intentions. In these twilight hours, every swipe of red lipstick is a stroke of mystery, adding to the enigma of the night and the allure of the woman who wears it. In Manhattan, where every evening is a tale waiting to unfold, the perfect red lip is the enchantress's most trusted ally.

Completed Tasks: Evening Enchantress Activities

Inspirational Quote

THE WORLD IS FULL OF MAGICAL THINGS PATIENTLY WAITING FOR OUR WITS TO GROW SHARPER. — Bertrand Russell

Action Items: Intentions and Thoughts

The Romantic Muse

In the enchanting canvas of Manhattan, where every moment pulsates with the possibility of romance, there emerges the Romantic Muse. She's a figure who captures the heart of the city's softer side, her presence a gentle yet profound echo of love and allure. In the quiet corners of moonlit streets, in the intimate spaces of cozy restaurants, her choice of red lipstick speaks not in bold declarations, but in tender, inviting whispers. It's here, under the star-studded sky, that the Romantic Muse weaves her spell, with shades of red that tell tales of love, longing, and the timeless dance of courtship.

- **The Sunset Kiss: Soft and Dreamy for Twilight Moments**. As the sky turns a rosy hue at sunset, a soft, warm shade of red mirrors the romance of the twilight hour. This color is perfect for those dreamy moments, evoking the gentle caress of the setting sun and the promise of a night filled with romance.

- **The Candlelight Coral: Glowing and Intimate for Dinner by Candlelight**. In the flickering glow of candlelight, a coral-red shade shines best. It's a hue that's both warm and inviting, creating an atmosphere of intimacy and warmth, ideal for deep conversations and shared glances across the table.

- **The Starry Night Scarlet: Passionate and Mesmerizing for Starlit Strolls**. For a romantic walk under the starry Manhattan sky, a deep scarlet brings a touch of passion. It's a color that mesmerizes, evoking the mystery and beauty of a night spent under the stars, hand in hand with a loved one.

- **The Vintage Rose: Elegant and Timeless for Classic Romance**. Reflecting the elegance of old-world romance, a vintage rose shade is perfect for moments that feel like they're out of a classic love story. This timeless hue resonates with the charm of historical Manhattan, from its grand old theaters to its storied hotels.

- **The Morning After Mauve: Subtle and Refreshing for New Beginnings.** For those soft, tender mornings after a night of romance, a mauve shade whispers of new beginnings. Gentle and understated, it reflects the freshness of a new day in the city, perfect for a leisurely breakfast in bed or a quiet coffee at a sidewalk cafe.
- **The Garden Party Pink: Cheerful and Blossoming for Daytime Rendezvous.** In the verdant settings of Manhattan's garden terraces, a bright pink red is the ideal choice. This cheerful, blossoming hue captures the essence of daytime romance, reminiscent of blooming flowers and the playful, sunny side of love.
- **The Midnight Berry: Deep and Enigmatic for Late Night Confessions.** As the night deepens, a berry-red tint suits the mood of intimate, late-night conversations. Rich and enigmatic, this shade is ideal for those moments of heartfelt confessions and shared secrets, under the watchful eyes of the city's twinkling lights.
- **The Whispering Wine: Rich and Mysterious for Secret Trysts.** In the dimly lit corners of upscale lounges, a wine-red lipstick is the perfect accompaniment. This rich, deep hue speaks of hidden glances and whispered promises, adding an air of mystery and allure to late-night rendezvous.

In the vast romantic landscape of Manhattan, the Romantic Muse finds her expression in the subtle yet powerful shades of red. Each color is a note in the symphony of love's narrative, from the soft warmth of a sunset kiss to the deep passion of a starry night. These hues are more than just lipstick; they're the tools of romance, painting each encounter with emotions and memories. In the city that never sleeps, the Romantic Muse's lips tell stories not just of love found, but of the everlasting pursuit of romance in the heart of Manhattan.

Completed Tasks: Romantic Muse Activities

Inspirational Quote

I ARISE FULL OF EAGERNESS AND ENERGY, KNOWING WELL WHAT ACHIEVEMENT LIES AHEAD OF ME. — Zane Grey

Action Items: Intentions and Thoughts

The Statement Maker

As Manhattan's skyline ignites with the dazzling lights of nightfall, it beckons the arrival of The Statement Maker. In this city of endless narratives, where every corner tells a story, some choose to speak louder than others. The Statement Maker is a formidable presence, turning heads not just with her striking attire but with the bold, unapologetic red gracing her lips. This isn't just a color; it's a declaration, a manifestation of confidence and charisma that echoes through the bustling streets and crowded rooms. In the grand theater of Manhattan, where the night is an endless possibility, her lipstick is the brush with which she paints her mark.

- **The Fire Engine Red: Vivid and Commanding for Bold Entrances**. In a shade that's as fearless as the city itself, fire engine red stands out in any crowd. It's the choice for those grand entrances, where the Statement Maker is not just seen, but noticed, her lips a vivid emblem of her daring spirit.
- **The Deep Ruby: Rich and Luxurious for Opulent Gatherings**. For the lavish parties and exclusive events, deep ruby red is the Statement Maker's ally. Rich, luxurious, and full of depth, it complements the sparkling jewels and elegant gowns, making a statement of refined luxury.
- **The Electric Crimson: Energetic and Provocative for Nightlife Adventures**. As the city dives into its electric nightlife, a shade of electric crimson captures its essence. Bold and provocative, this red is for those vibrant nights of dance, music, and uninhibited fun, embodying the city's pulsating energy.
- **The Matte Scarlet: Chic and Modern for Trendsetting Moments**. In the trendy spots where the city's fashionistas gather, matte scarlet makes its mark. Chic, contemporary, and fashion-

forward, it's a shade for the modern Statement Maker, one who sets trends rather than follows them.

- **The Classic Hollywood Red: Timeless and Glamorous for Star-Studded Events.** For occasions that call for timeless glamour, the classic Hollywood red is the Statement Maker's go-to. This iconic, glamorous shade harkens back to the golden age of cinema, perfect for moments that demand a touch of classic, old-world charm in the modern Manhattan setting.
- **The Metallic Rose: Edgy and Reflective for Artistic Gatherings.** At art openings and creative gatherings, a metallic rose red stands out. This edgy, reflective shade is a nod to the city's innovative art scene, capturing the light and the imagination in equal measure, perfect for the Statement Maker who's also a patron of the arts.
- **The Bold Burgundy: Deep and Mysterious for Intimate Soirees.** In the more intimate settings of private soirees or exclusive clubs, a bold burgundy makes a profound statement. It's a deep, mysterious shade that speaks of sophistication and a certain je ne sais quoi, ideal for the Statement Maker who prefers to intrigue and captivate.

In the ever-evolving narrative of Manhattan, the Statement Maker's choice of red lipstick stands as a bold punctuation. Each shade is a chapter in her story, a testament to her strength, her flair, and her unwavering presence. In a city where being bold is the only way to be, these reds are more than mere accents; they are symbols of the audacity and glamour that pulse through the veins of Manhattan. For the Statement Maker, every night is a canvas, and her lipstick, a color with which to paint her indelible mark on the city's endless tale.

Completed Tasks: Statement Maker Activities

Inspirational Quote

WITH SELF-DISCIPLINE MOST ANYTHING IS POSSIBLE. — Theodore Roosevelt

Action Items: Intentions and Thoughts

Action Items: Intentions and Thoughts

Central Park Chic: Natural Looks that Dazzle in the Daylight

Manhattan, a city where the line between the cosmopolitan and the organic beautifully blurs. Here, amid the hum of traffic and the whispers of ancient trees, each step you take is a symphony of old-world charm and modern-day flair. It's not merely about reaching your destination, but about the elegance and authenticity with which you present yourself along the journey.

Imagine: Strolling through Central Park on a sunny afternoon, the golden light filtering through the leaves, casting a gentle glow on your face. The world doesn't see you draped in the latest couture, but is instead entranced by the natural radiance of your complexion. That, darling, is Central Park Chic, a canvas of subtlety, where less is always more.

In this refreshing chapter of The Manhattan Diaries, we unveil the allure of the natural. From the dew-kissed flush of morning freshness to the soft shimmer of a sunlit glow, you'll unravel the art of enhancing your inherent beauty, celebrating your individuality.

But this isn't just a superficial dance with cosmetics—far from it. It's about harmonizing with the essence of the city, tapping into the serene beauty of its green heart, Central Park. It's about the juxtaposition of skyscrapers and verdant landscapes, and reflecting that balance on your visage.

So, journey with me through tree-lined pathways and alongside tranquil lakes. Let's discover beauty secrets whispered by the wind and endorsed by the sun. In Manhattan, where nature and neon entwine, every gaze towards the mirror is a reflection of the city's dual spirit. Ready to embrace the natural, the raw, the real? The Manhattan Diaries beckons, where your look is as refreshing as a Central Park spring morning.

The Dewy Dawn Look

In the heart of Manhattan, where the city that never sleeps surrenders to the gentle embrace of dawn, a new kind of magic unfolds—the Dewy Dawn Look. It's a signature style that captures the essence of a fresh beginning, an awakening of the senses, and the promise of a brand-new day. As the sun paints the skyline with its first rays, Manhattan's elite embark on their daily rituals to unveil a look that exudes radiance and vitality. Join me as we uncover the secrets behind this ethereal morning transformation, one step at a time.

- **The Morning Glow Ritual**. Before the City stirs, Manhattan's beauty aficionados embark on their quest for a flawless complexion. The Dewy Dawn Look begins with a skincare regimen designed to hydrate and illuminate. Serums, moisturizers, and facial mists come together to create a radiant canvas that seems to catch the first light of dawn.
- **The Subtle Sparkle of Eye Makeup**. To accentuate the eyes without overwhelming the natural beauty of the morning, a soft and understated eye makeup approach is key. A touch of champagne or rose gold eyeshadow, complemented by a swipe of mascara and well-groomed brows, adds a subtle sparkle that mirrors the cityscape.
- **Rosy Flush of Blush**. The Dewy Dawn Look thrives on the flush of youth, and what better way to achieve it than with a gentle application of rosy blush? Manhattan's style mavens understand the art of blush placement, using it to accentuate their cheekbones and bring out their inner radiance.
- **The Luminous Lip**. A sheer and dewy lip balm or gloss in shades of soft pink or peach completes the look. It adds a touch of freshness and vibrancy to the lips, making them ready for the day's encounters, whether it's a business meeting or a casual coffee date.

- **Hair That Breathes**. To complement the Dewy Dawn Look, Manhattan's elite opt for effortlessly tousled or lightly waved hair that seems to dance in the morning breeze. It's a style that exudes ease and sophistication, perfect for navigating the city's early hours.
- **Morning Meditation**. Manhattan's trendsetters often kickstart their day with a moment of mindfulness. Whether it's a quick meditation session or some deep breathing exercises, finding inner peace is an essential part of the Dewy Dawn routine.
- **Wardrobe Magic**. Dressing for the Dewy Dawn Look means selecting outfits that are comfortable yet effortlessly chic. Light, breathable fabrics and pastel hues are often the choice to complement the overall morning glow.
- **Fresh-Faced Confidence**. The Dewy Dawn Look is not just about makeup; it's about confidence. Manhattan's elite understand that true beauty radiates from within, and their morning routine is a celebration of self assuredness.
- **Scent of Success**. Fragrance is a final touch that should not be underestimated. A light, floral or citrusy scent adds a subtle layer of sophistication to the Dewy Dawn Look, leaving a memorable impression wherever they go.

The Dewy Dawn Look is a tribute to the quiet elegance of morning in Manhattan. It's for the woman who finds beauty in simplicity, who steps out into the day not to overpower but to harmonize with the world around her. This look is an embrace of the new day, a celebration of fresh starts, and a reflection of the city's quiet morning beauty. In a place where every day holds endless potential, this look is a reminder that sometimes, the most profound statement is one of serene simplicity.

Completed Tasks: Dewy Dawn Look Activities

Inspirational Quote

OF ALL THINGS VISIBLE, THE HIGHEST IS THE HEAVEN OF THE FIXED STARS. — Nicolaus Copernicus

Action Items: Intentions and Thoughts

Sun-Kissed and Subtle

Darlings, let's talk about the enchanting world of the Sun-Kissed and Subtle look. It's the kind of beauty that whispers rather than shouts, the kind that makes you look effortlessly radiant, as if you've just strolled through a sunlit garden. In the bustling heart of Manhattan, where the pace is as fast as the city lights are bright, there's something utterly captivating about embracing a look that's soft, understated, and utterly elegant. It's a look favored by the city's elite, those who understand that less can indeed be more. So, pour yourself a cup of herbal tea, and let's dive into the secrets of this effortlessly chic Manhattan style.

- **Barely There Makeup**. The Sun-Kissed and Subtle look begins with makeup that celebrates your natural beauty. It's about creating a flawless complexion with a dewy finish that makes your skin look like it's been bathed in sunlight. You'll want to keep things minimal here—think a touch of blush to bring out your cheeks' natural flush, a soft eyeshadow that enhances your eyes without being overly dramatic, and a nude lip color that accentuates your lips' natural shape. This makeup is like a gentle enhancement, emphasizing your best features without covering up who you truly are.

- **Soft, Natural Hair**. Your hairstyle plays a pivotal role in achieving the Sun-Kissed and Subtle look. Loose waves that cascade gracefully down your shoulders or a simple yet sleek ponytail are both excellent choices. The key here is to keep things natural and unforced. The hairstyle should appear as if you woke up with your hair looking this beautiful, effortlessly chic.

- **Neutral Tones**. When it comes to your wardrobe, think of a palette that mirrors the softness and elegance of this style. Beige, soft pink, pale gold, and muted earthy tones are your best friends. These colors exude sophistication and class without overpowering your overall look. The idea is to embrace a neutral canvas that allows your natural beauty to take center stage.

- **Sun-Kissed Glow**. To truly capture that sun-kissed essence, a touch of bronzer or highlighter can work wonders. Apply it delicately to areas where the sun naturally hits your face—the high points of your cheekbones, the bridge of your nose, and your brow bones. This creates a luminous glow that gives the impression of sun-kissed skin, as if you've just returned from a weekend getaway in a coastal paradise.
- **Minimal Accessories**. Less is indeed more in the world of the Sun-Kissed and Subtle look. Instead of loading up on accessories, opt for a minimalist approach. Delicate jewelry or perhaps one statement piece can add that touch of elegance without overwhelming your appearance. The goal here is to achieve an effortless and understated chic that radiates confidence.
- **Effortless Daytime Glam**. The Sun-Kissed and Subtle look is perfect for daytime events, such as brunches, garden parties, or strolls through Central Park. It's all about feeling glamorous without appearing overdressed. Your makeup should have a dewy finish that's fresh and radiant, reflecting the natural sunlight.

In the heart of Manhattan, where the city that never sleeps surrenders to the gentle embrace of dawn, a new kind of magic unfolds—the Dewy Dawn Look. It's a signature style that captures the essence of a fresh beginning, an awakening of the senses, and the promise of a brand-new day. As the sun paints the skyline with its first rays, Manhattan's elite embark on their daily rituals to unveil a look that exudes radiance and vitality. Join me as we uncover the secrets behind this ethereal morning transformation, one step at a time.

Completed Tasks: Sun-Kissed and Subtle Activities

Inspirational Quote

THINK WITH YOUR WHOLE BODY. — Taisen Deshimaru

Action Items: Intentions and Thoughts

The Flush of Nature

In the heart of Manhattan, where the urban jungle meets the lush oasis of Central Park, a distinct beauty trend has emerged—the Flush of Nature. It's a makeup look that effortlessly captures the rosy, healthy glow of a leisurely stroll through the park on a crisp autumn day. As Manhattan's elite know, this look is all about embracing the natural allure of flushed cheeks and subtle, earthy tones. Join me as we explore the secrets behind The Flush of Nature, a look that embodies the enchanting harmony between the city that never sleeps and the tranquility of nature.

- **Effortlessly Rosy Cheeks**. The key to The Flush of Nature lies in achieving rosy cheeks that appear as if you've just returned from a brisk walk in Central Park. It starts with a delicate application of a cream blush in soft, warm shades such as peach, rose, or coral. The goal is to mimic the subtle flush that naturally graces your cheeks when exposed to the brisk Manhattan air.

- **Minimalist Base**. Manhattan's elite understand that less is often more. The Flush of Nature calls for a minimalist approach to your base makeup. A lightweight, dewy foundation or tinted moisturizer that allows your skin's natural texture to shine through is the foundation of this look.

- **Earthy Tones and Subtle Highlights**. To accentuate the natural beauty of the Flush of Nature, earthy eyeshadows in warm browns and soft taupes are applied to the eyelids. Subtle highlights are used sparingly on the high points of the face, providing a gentle luminosity that mimics the soft sunlight filtering through the trees in Central Park.

- **Glossy Lips**. Keep your lip color understated yet inviting with a glossy finish. Opt for shades like soft pinks, nudes, or even a hint of berry to enhance your lips' natural color. This adds a touch of allure without overpowering the overall look.

- **Dewy Skin Finish**. Achieving that fresh, dewy complexion is essential for The Flush of Nature. Manhattan's elite swear by hydrating setting sprays or facial mists to lock in moisture and give their skin a radiant, just-exercised glow.
- **Natural Brows**. The brows play a crucial role in this look. Keep them well-groomed and use a brow gel to lightly define and set them in place. The goal is to maintain a soft, natural arch that frames your face elegantly.
- **Sun-Kissed Freckles**. Embrace your natural freckles or create faux freckles with a light brown or taupe eyeliner pencil. Gently dot them across your cheeks and nose for that youthful, sun-kissed effect.
- **Subtle Mascara**. For your lashes, a coat of brown mascara adds definition without the drama of jet-black mascara. It complements the earthy tones of the Flush of Nature while keeping the focus on your rosy cheeks and glowing skin.
- **Softly Defined Eyes**. Complete The Flush of Nature by softly defining the eyes with a thin line of brown or taupe eyeliner. This adds just enough definition to enhance your natural eye shape without overshadowing the gentle, earthy tones of the overall look.

As you embrace the Flush of Nature, you'll discover that it's not just a makeup trend; it's a lifestyle. It's about connecting with the beauty of nature while confidently striding through the bustling streets of Manhattan. With this look, you'll effortlessly blend the tranquility of Central Park with the vibrant energy of the city. So, next time you're strolling through the heart of Manhattan, let The Flush of Nature be your signature, a reflection of your inner elegance and connection to the world around you.

Completed Tasks: Flush of Nature Activities

Inspirational Quote

GRACE IS THE BEAUTY OF FORM UNDER THE INFLUENCE OF FREEDOM. — Friedrich Schiller

Action Items: Intentions and Thoughts

Barely-There Beauty

In the bustling streets of Manhattan, where the energy is electric and the pace is relentless, the Barely-There Beauty look has become a timeless favorite among the city's elite. It's the kind of understated elegance that effortlessly blends into the urban landscape while leaving a lasting impression. This style is all about embracing your natural beauty, enhancing your best features, and letting your inner radiance shine through. In this chapter of "City-Slick Glamour," we'll unravel the secrets to achieving this effortlessly chic look that's perfect for every Manhattanite.

- **Flawless Skin Foundation**. The key to the Barely-There Beauty look is a flawless complexion that appears almost untouched. Start with a lightweight, sheer foundation or tinted moisturizer that evens out your skin tone while allowing your natural beauty to peek through. The goal is to achieve a fresh, healthy glow without heavy coverage.
- **Minimalist Makeup**. Less is more when it comes to makeup. Opt for neutral and nude shades for your eyeshadow, blush, and lipstick. Soft beige or peach tones work wonders to enhance your features while keeping the look understated. A touch of nude lip gloss adds a hint of shine without overpowering.
- **Effortless Eyebrows**. Well-groomed brows frame your face and are crucial for this look. Use a brow pencil or powder that matches your natural brow color to define and shape them slightly. The goal is to maintain a natural and effortless arch that complements your features.
- **Subtle Eyeliner**. Skip the dramatic winged eyeliner and instead, apply a thin line of brown or taupe eyeliner along your upper lash line. This subtle definition enhances your eyes without drawing too much attention.

- **Mascara Magic**. A coat of brown mascara is all you need to give your lashes a subtle lift. Brown mascara adds depth to your lashes while maintaining the Barely-There Beauty look's soft and understated allure.
- **Fresh-Faced Blush**. Opt for a cream blush in a soft, rosy hue. Apply it to the apples of your cheeks and blend it out for a natural flush of color. This step adds a healthy glow to your complexion, reminiscent of a brisk morning walk in Central Park.
- **Natural Hair**. To complement your minimalistic makeup, go for relaxed, natural-looking hair. Soft waves or a low bun are perfect choices. The key is to keep your hairstyle effortless and in harmony with your Barely-There Beauty makeup.
- **Radiant Confidence**. The most important element of the Barely-There Beauty look is confidence. Embrace your natural beauty, carry yourself with poise, and let your inner radiance shine through. In Manhattan, where the city's pulse is relentless, this look is a testament to the power of understated elegance.
- **Sheer Lip Tint**. Enhance your lips with just a touch of color using a sheer lip tint. Choose a shade that closely matches your natural lip color for a subtle enhancement that complements the Barely-There Beauty ethos. This simple addition keeps your lips looking healthy and plump, adding to the overall minimalistic yet polished appearance.

In a city that never sleeps, the Barely-There Beauty look is a nod to the beauty of simplicity and the allure of authenticity. It's a style that says, "I'm here, and I'm confident in my own skin." So, Manhattanites, embrace this timeless look and let your inner beauty steal the spotlight in the city that never stops shining.

Completed Tasks: Barely-There Beauty Activities

Inspirational Quote

IN A GENTLE WAY, YOU CAN SHAKE THE WORLD. — Mahatma Gandhi

Action Items: Intentions and Thoughts

Action Items: Intentions and Thoughts

Broadway's Blushing Beauties: Achieving Cheeks that Pop and Highlight

Manhattan, the very heart where dreams are sung, danced, and draped in dazzling lights. This city doesn't just witness performances; it lives and breathes them, with every gesture, every note, every shade thrown by the setting sun against its towers of dreams. In this metropolis of endless acts, life isn't just about being seen; it's about making a mark—with drama, elegance, and that undeniable Broadway flair.

Now, picture this: You're floating down the Theater District, and while the marquees shine bright, you rival their luminescence. It's not the designer ensemble that captivates the crowd, but the drama and depth of your cheeks, contoured and highlighted to perfection. That, my dear, is the Broadway Glow, an artistry that tells tales of passion, drama, and a lifetime of curtain calls.

In this tantalizing chapter of The Manhattan Diaries, we dive into the world of stage-ready radiance. From the soft, romantic hues of a leading lady in love to the fierce, fiery shades of a diva taking charge, you'll learn to accentuate every emotion with just a sweep of a brush.

But Broadway isn't just about the bright lights and bold choices—no. It's about resonating with the pulse of the city, feeling the heartbeat of every love story, tragedy, and triumph that graces its stages. Embracing the highs and the lows, mastering the chiaroscuro of Manhattan's dynamic life.

So, accompany me, as we waltz through backstage secrets and front row marvels. As we paint our faces with tales of love, desire, laughter, and a few tears. Because in Manhattan, every glance, every smile, every blush is a story waiting to be told. Darling, the spotlight is on, and the city is your audience. Step into The Manhattan Diaries—where your glow rivals the city's brightest star.

The Dramatic Contour

In the dazzling world of Manhattan, where every corner is a stage and every day a performance, dramatic contouring is more than just makeup-it's an art. Picture this: You're standing in the bustling Theater District, surrounded by the glamour of Broadway. Your makeup isn't just a mere cosmetic application; it's a statement. The sharp angles of your contoured cheeks rival the drama of the stage, casting shadows and highlights that command attention. This, my dear, is the Dramatic Contour, a masterpiece of light and shadow that tells a story of allure, sophistication, and an unapologetic love for the spotlight.

- **Achieving the Perfect Drama: The Art of Sculpting**. Contouring isn't just about covering up imperfections; it's about enhancing your natural beauty. Learn the delicate art of sculpting your face, creating shadows and definition that rival the city's skyline. It's a canvas, and your face is the masterpiece.
- **Choosing the Right Shades**. The key to a flawless dramatic contour lies in selecting the perfect contouring and highlighting shades for your unique skin tone. Delve into the secrets of shade selection, ensuring that every stroke of your brush contributes to the captivating allure.
- **Blending Like a Pro**. Mastery of the art of blending is your ticket to achieving that seamless, chiseled look that captures the essence of Manhattan's allure. Dive into the techniques of blending, where contrasting shades come together harmoniously, ensuring your contours are as sharp as the city's skyscrapers.
- **Enhancing Your Features**. Contouring isn't a one-size-fits-all approach. Discover how to tailor your contouring to your unique features, from accentuating the sharp angles of your cheekbones to

defining the slender line of your jaw. Each stroke enhances your natural beauty, telling a story as captivating as the city itself.

- **The Power of Lighting**. Learn the tricks of the trade when it comes to using lighting to your advantage. Whether it's the soft glow of a dressing room mirror or the dazzling stage lights, understanding how different lighting conditions can affect your contour is key to mastering this art.
- **Blurring the Lines**. Discover how to create a flawless transition between your contoured areas and the rest of your makeup. Blurring the lines ensures that your contour looks seamless and natural, even when you're under the spotlight.
- **Long-Lasting Drama**. Explore techniques and products that can help your dramatic contour stay in place throughout a long evening of performances, parties, and city adventures. Your makeup should be as enduring as your love for Manhattan's nightlife.
- **Contouring Beyond the Stage**. While dramatic contouring is a must for Broadway beauties, it's a versatile skill that can enhance your everyday look as you navigate the streets of Manhattan. Learn how to adapt your contouring techniques for various occasions, from matinee shows to late-night dinners at the city's finest restaurants.

In the world of Manhattan, where every day is a performance and the city's heartbeat is an applause, your makeup becomes your costume, your face a canvas. As you step into the spotlight, remember: with dramatic contouring, you're not just making an entrance; you're stealing the show. Welcome to The Manhattan Diaries, where your face becomes a work of art as iconic as the city itself.

Completed Tasks: Dramatic Contour Activities

Inspirational Quote

IF WE DID ALL THE THINGS, WE ARE CAPABLE OF, WE WOULD LITERALLY ASTOUND OURSELVES. — Thomas A. Edison

Action Items: Intentions and Thoughts

Radiant Highlights

In the dazzling world of Manhattan, where every street corner holds the promise of a star-studded encounter, it's not just about being seen—it's about basking in your own radiant glow. Picture this: You're stepping out of a swanky rooftop bar, the city lights shimmering in the background, and your skin is aglow with the radiance of a thousand stars. That, my dear, is the Radiant Highlight—a makeup technique that elevates your beauty to celestial heights.

- **Luminous from Within**. Discover the art of creating a radiant, lit-from-within complexion that mimics the natural glow of Manhattan's city lights. From the high points of your cheekbones to the bridge of your nose, learn how to strategically apply highlighter for a luminous effect that turns heads wherever you go.
- **Sculpting with Light**. Explore the magic of light and shadow as you sculpt your face to perfection. Highlighter isn't just about illumination; it's a tool for defining your features. Find out how to contour with light, emphasizing your best assets and creating a three-dimensional allure that captivates the city's elite.
- **The Secrets of Strobing**. Dive into the world of strobing, a technique beloved by Manhattan's fashionistas and socialites. Strobing is all about amplifying your natural radiance; make sure to master this technique with finesse. From choosing the right highlighter shade to placement that catches the light just so, you'll be a strobing sensation.
- **Day to Night Brilliance**. Transition your radiant highlights from daytime chic to evening glamour as effortlessly as you transition from brunch to Broadway. Learn the secrets of touch-ups and layering that keep your glow alive from sunrise to the city's glittering skyline.

- **The Power of Layering**. Delve into the world of layering your highlighter for a multi-dimensional effect that evolves throughout the day and night. Discover how to apply creams and powders strategically to achieve a look that's as dynamic as the city itself.
- **Highlighting for Your Face Shape**. Understand that not all highlighter techniques are one-size-fits-all. Let this understanding guide you in choosing the right highlighting methods for your unique face shape, enhancing your features in harmony with Manhattan's diverse landscape.
- **Mastering the Ethereal Glow**. Elevate your highlighter game to a celestial level by exploring advanced techniques that create an ethereal, otherworldly radiance. Whether you're attending a rooftop gala or a late-night jazz club, you'll enchant with your otherworldly glow.
- **Customizing Your Canvas**. Tailor your highlighting to suit the seasons of Manhattan, from the bright summer sun to the subtle winter light. Adjust the intensity and shades of your highlighter to reflect the ambient light of each season, ensuring your skin always looks its best, no matter the weather or occasion.
- **Glowing Recommendations**. Uncover the top picks for highlighters from beauty insiders and makeup professionals. Get the scoop on the best products for achieving a radiant highlight, whether you're looking for a subtle sheen or a bold, glamorous shimmer.

Radiant highlights aren't just makeup; they're an art form. They're your personal spotlight, and they shine brightest against the backdrop of Manhattan's cosmopolitan wonder. Join us as we unravel the mysteries of luminosity, from the glow of a Broadway marquee to the sparkle of a champagne flute at an upscale soiree. Welcome to The Manhattan Diaries, where you're the star of your own radiant show.

Completed Tasks: Radiant Highlights Activities

Inspirational Quote

OUR LIFE IS WHAT OUR THOUGHTS MAKE IT. — Marcus Aurelius

Action Items: Intentions and Thoughts

Rosy Blush

Manhattan, a city where every sidewalk is a catwalk, and every moment is an opportunity to shine. In this bustling metropolis, where the avenues are your runways, the theaters your stages, and the galleries your exhibitions, your look must always be on point. Amongst the towering skyscrapers and buzzing street corners, one thing remains constant—the allure of a perfectly flushed cheek, the embodiment of rosy health and timeless sophistication.

- **The Art of Rosy Elegance**. Dive into the world of rosy blush, and experiment with the delicate balance between a natural flush and an artful statement. Then, choose the right shade and texture to match your style, whether you're strolling through Central Park or attending a high-society gala.
- **The City's Blushing Secrets**. Uncover the insider tips and tricks used by Manhattan's elite to achieve that coveted rosy glow. From the Upper East Side to the West Village, each neighborhood has its own take on this timeless look. Hop on a journey through the city's unique blush trends, helping you find the one that resonates with your inner New Yorker.
- **Sculpting with Rosy Hues**. Blush isn't just about adding color to your cheeks; it's about sculpting and defining your features. Use blush strategically to highlight your bone structure and create a radiant, contoured effect that's both modern and classic.
- **Day to Night Blushing**. Explore versatile techniques that seamlessly transition your daytime blush into a sultry evening look. Whether you're heading to a business meeting or a glamorous cocktail party, your blush will adapt to every scene, just like a Manhattanite.

- **Iconic Blushing Moments**. Explore the history of rosy blush in Manhattan, from its origins in the early 20th century to the present day. Learn how legendary Manhattan women like Audrey Hepburn and Marilyn Monroe embraced the power of rosy cheeks to define their signature looks.
- **The Modern Manhattan Blush Wardrobe**. Discover the essential blush products and tools every Manhattanite needs in her makeup arsenal. From cream blushes for a dewy daytime look to powder blushes for a sophisticated evening appearance, building a versatile collection along the way.
- **Blush Etiquette and Social Significance**. In Manhattan, the subtle nuances of makeup can carry significant social weight. Explore the unspoken rules and etiquette surrounding blush application, from boardroom meetings to exclusive society soirees.
- **Blush as a Statement**. Uncover how Manhattan's fashion-forward individuals use rosy blush as a statement piece, complementing their outfits and conveying their personality. From minimalist chic to bold and audacious, use blush to express your unique style in the city that never sleeps.
- **Seasonal Rosy Trends**. Embrace the changing seasons of Manhattan with blush tones that reflect the city's dynamic palette. Adapt your blush color to suit the crispness of fall, the freshness of spring, the warmth of summer, and the coolness of winter, ensuring your look remains harmoniously in step with nature.

Your rosy blush isn't just a makeup choice; it's a reflection of your inner Manhattan mystique. Join us as we journey through the city's streets, unveiling the secrets of rosy perfection that have graced the faces of the most iconic Manhattan women. Welcome to The Manhattan Diaries, where your blush is your signature, and the city is your canvas.

Completed Tasks: Blush Sculpting Activities

Inspirational Quote

ALL YOU NEED IS THE PLAN, THE ROAD MAP, AND THE COURAGE TO PRESS ON TO YOUR DESTINATION. — Earl Nightingale

Action Items: Intentions and Thoughts

Blend and Buff

Manhattan, the island of dreams, where every passerby could be a potential admirer, and every street corner a stage waiting for your performance. In this city that never sleeps, makeup is your trusted ally, the artistry that transforms you from a spectator to the star of your own show. The streets are your runway, and every sidewalk your red carpet, so let's delve into the art of blending and buffing, where your face becomes the canvas for a masterpiece that tells the world, "I've arrived."

- **The Art of Blending**. Manhattan's elite understand that the secret to a flawless complexion lies in mastering the art of blending. Discover the techniques and products that will help you achieve a seamless, airbrushed finish that can withstand the city's demands, from dawn till dusk.
- **Tools of the Trade**. From makeup brushes to sponges and beyond, explore the essential tools that Manhattan's beauty connoisseurs rely on. Learn how to choose the right brushes and perfect your application skills to achieve a professional-level look.
- **Contouring and Highlighting Mastery**. Contouring and highlighting are the magic wands of makeup artistry, capable of sculpting your face and bestowing a radiant glow. Whether you're aiming for chiseled cheekbones fit for the runway or a luminous complexion that rivals the city lights, we'll guide you through these transformative techniques.
- **The Manhattan Makeup Wardrobe**. Makeup in Manhattan isn't just a routine; it's a reflection of personal style. Explore the must-have products that should grace every Manhattanite's vanity, from foundation to setting spray. Your makeup wardrobe is your arsenal for conquering the city with confidence.

- **The Flawless Finish**. Achieving a flawless complexion is the cornerstone of Manhattan's makeup scene. Learn the secrets to selecting the right foundation shade, texture, and finish to create a base that looks as impeccable in natural daylight as it does under the city's dazzling lights.
- **Day to Night Transition**. Manhattan's vibrant lifestyle often demands a quick transformation from daytime chic to nighttime glamour. Experiment with the tips and tricks to seamlessly transition your makeup look, so you're ready to shine at cocktail parties, galas, or a spontaneous night out in the city.
- **Setting the Stage**. Setting sprays and powders are your allies in ensuring your makeup stays in place, no matter what the city throws your way. Explore the products and techniques that will lock in your makeup, so you can confidently navigate Manhattan's bustling streets.
- **Personalized Beauty**. In the melting pot of Manhattan, individuality is celebrated. Tailor your makeup routine to highlight your unique features and personality, making your look truly your own amidst the diverse tapestry of the city.
- **Texture Techniques**. Master the interplay of textures, from matte to shimmer, to enhance your makeup's visual impact; blending different finishes can add depth and dimension to your look, perfectly capturing the dynamic multifaceted spirit of Manhattan.

In Manhattan, where every corner holds a new adventure, makeup is your passport to self-expression and allure. Join us on this journey into the world of blending and buffing, where your face becomes a canvas for artistry. In The Manhattan Diaries, blending and buffing are the first strokes in your masterpiece, setting the stage for a captivating performance in the city that never ceases to inspire.

Completed Tasks: Blend and Buff Activities

Inspirational Quote

VITALITY SHOWS IN NOT ONLY THE ABILITY TO PERSIST BUT THE ABILITY TO START OVER. — F. Scott Fitzgerald

Action Items: Intentions and Thoughts

Action Items: Intentions and Thoughts

The Wall Street Wing: Eyeliners that Mean Business

Manhattan, where ambition isn't just a buzzword—it's the lifeblood, coursing through the very veins of its avenues. This city doesn't simply observe the daily hustle—it's entwined in it, with every deal sealed and every risk taken, echoing tales of power moves, sharp instincts, and an audacity that knows no bounds. Here, in the heart of commerce, it's not just about sealing the deal; it's about doing so with a flair that turns heads, in the boardroom and beyond.

Picture this: You're navigating the maze of Wall Street, where titans roam and futures are determined. But today, it's not your portfolio that's drawing attention, or the sharpness of your suit—it's the fierce precision of your eyeliner, declaring to the world that you mean business. This, darling, is the Wall Street Wing, a signature that speaks of power, prowess, and an unyielding spirit.

In this captivating chapter of The Manhattan Diaries, we delve deep into the allure of the perfect winged eyeliner. From the demure hint that suggests a savvy investor to the bold, unapologetic swoop of a Wall Street maverick, learn the art and technique behind each stroke that resonates with ambition.

But it's not just about the aesthetics—oh no. It's a reflection of the relentless tempo of finance, the strategy behind every trade, the vision behind every venture. It's about capturing the essence of Manhattan's financial district, where every gaze, every flutter, every blink can change fortunes.

Come with me, as we master the strokes and sweeps that aren't just about enhancing the eyes, but capturing the spirit of a world where risk and reward dance in tandem. Because in Manhattan, especially on Wall Street, every look is a statement, every wing an emblem of ambition. Ready yourself, for the city is watching, and it's your time to captivate. Dive into The Manhattan Diaries—where your gaze can be as formidable as your portfolio.

The Subtle Statement

In the bustling corridors of Wall Street, where power suits and sharp minds set the scene, there's a subtle yet potent form of expression—the Subtle Statement eyeliner. It's a look that speaks volumes in hushed tones, a minimalist stroke that mirrors the understated confidence of Manhattan's financial mavens. In a world where every detail is scrutinized, the Subtle Statement is the perfect embodiment of power, precision, and poise. It's for the woman who understands that in the high-stakes game of finance, sometimes the most impactful statements are made with the slightest flourish.

- **The Sleek Line: Precision and Poise**. Opt for a thin, precise line that hugs the lash line. This sleek application symbolizes the accuracy and sharp focus required in the world of finance. It's a look that's professional, polished, and subtly commanding.
- **The Soft Wing: A Hint of Ambition**. Add a small, soft wing at the outer corner of the eye. This slight extension is a nod to the ambitious spirit of Wall Street, suggesting a readiness to take calculated risks. It's understated yet suggests a forward-thinking attitude.
- **The Matte Finish: Subdued Sophistication**. Choose a matte eyeliner for its understated elegance. A non-glossy finish is key to this look, as it eschews overt glamour in favor of a more subdued, sophisticated form of chic, resonating with the professional ambiance of the financial district.
- **The Neutral Palette: Blending In to Stand Out**. Complement the eyeliner with neutral eyeshadows. Shades of taupe, beige, or soft browns underscore the Subtle Statement's ethos of sophistication without overstatement.

- **The Minimalist Touch: Less is More**. Embrace the minimalist approach by keeping the rest of your makeup understated. A light foundation, a touch of nude or soft pink lipstick, and a hint of mascara complement the Subtle Statement eyeliner. This approach reflects the Wall Street ethos of efficiency and effectiveness, where every element serves a purpose.
- **The Soft Smudge: Subtly Defined Edges**. For a softer look, slightly smudge the eyeliner at the edges. This technique adds a hint of depth without overwhelming the eye, symbolizing the adaptability and nuanced understanding necessary in the financial world. It's a small but impactful adjustment that softens the look while maintaining its intention.
- **The Understated Elegance: Quality Over Quantity**. Choose a high-quality eyeliner that guarantees a smooth application and lasting wear. The emphasis on quality over quantity resonates with the Wall Street principle of valuing substance over flashiness, ensuring your Subtle Statement remains impeccable throughout the day's challenges.

In the world of Wall Street, where every decision can tip the scales, the Subtle Statement eyeliner is more than a makeup choice; it's a strategic tool. It exemplifies the power of understatement in an environment where boldness is the norm. This eyeliner style is a testament to the wearer's confidence and acumen, a subtle symbol of her ability to navigate the complexities of finance with grace and precision. It's not just a look, but a statement of one's approach to the world of high finance—calculated, confident, and strikingly effective.

Completed Tasks: Subtle Statement Activities

Inspirational Quote

WHEN THE SUN IS SHINING, I CAN DO ANYTHING; NO MOUNTAIN IS TOO HIGH, NO TROUBLE TOO DIFFICULT TO OVERCOME. — Wilma Rudolph

Action Items: Intentions and Thoughts

The Bold Boardroom Look

In the high-powered boardrooms of Manhattan, where decisions shape futures and the stakes are sky-high, there emerges a look that commands respect and exudes confidence—the Bold Boardroom Look. This isn't just a makeup style; it's a statement of authority, a declaration of one's presence in the demanding world of business. Here, the eyeliner isn't just a part of your ensemble; it's an extension of your professional persona, a bold stroke that says you're not just in the room, you're leading it. For the woman who navigates the corridors of power with ease, the Bold Boardroom Look is her armor and her strength.

- **The Statement Wing: Defining Leadership**. Opt for a bold winged eyeliner that extends confidently beyond the outer corner of the eye. This striking look embodies leadership and determination, mirroring the assertiveness required to take the lead in high-stakes discussions and negotiations.
- **The Intense Color: Depth and Boldness**. Choose a deep, richly pigmented eyeliner. A jet black or dark brown provides the intensity needed to underline your words with visual impact. It's about making your gaze as compelling as your insights and arguments.
- **The Thick Line: Unapologetic Presence**. A thicker line above the lash line asserts your presence. It's a visual cue that aligns with the boldness of your ideas and the strength of your convictions. This look is unapologetic, much like the business acumen required in the boardroom.
- **The Polished Finish: Sleek and Professional**. Ensure the eyeliner is impeccably applied with a smooth, polished finish. No smudges or uneven lines—it's about precision and perfection, reflecting the attention to detail and meticulousness necessary in corporate decision-making.

- **The Seamless Blend: Balanced and Dynamic**. Incorporate a subtle eyeshadow blend into your look to add dimension without diminishing the impact of the bold eyeliner. Choose neutral or matte shades that enhance the eyeliner's boldness, creating a balanced yet dynamic eye makeup that resonates with the multifaceted nature of boardroom dynamics.
- **The Confident Lower Lash Line: Subtle Definition**. To complete the bold look, add a touch of eyeliner on the lower lash line, but keep it softer and more subdued. This adds definition to the eyes without overpowering the upper lid's statement, maintaining a confident and focused look that's perfect for direct eye contact during important discussions.
- **The Impeccable Brow: Framing the Vision**. Give attention to your eyebrows as they frame your bold eyeliner look. Well-groomed and defined brows contribute to the overall impression of confidence and control. This echoes the precision and attention to detail that are hallmarks of a successful boardroom leader.
- **Strategic Highlighting: A Touch of Brilliance**. Enhance the impact of your bold eyeliner by placing a small amount of highlighter at the inner corners of your eyes and just below the brow bone.

In the world of high finance and corporate strategy, the Bold Boardroom Look is more than just makeup; it's a part of your strategic toolkit. This eyeliner style resonates with the energy of Manhattan's business district, a reflection of the ambition, power, and unyielding determination that fuels the city's corporate warriors. It's for the woman who steps into the boardroom not just to participate, but to dominate; not just to speak, but to be heard. In this environment, where every detail counts, your eyeliner is as crucial as the figures in your presentation—bold, precise, and undeniably powerful.

Completed Tasks: Bold Boardroom Look Activities

Inspirational Quote

HOW GLORIOUS A GREETING THE SUN GIVES THE MOUNTAINS! — John Muir

Action Items: Intentions and Thoughts

The After-Hours Edge

As the sun sets over the Manhattan skyline, the city's heartbeat shifts, signaling the transition from corporate precision to after-hours elegance. It's in this twilight zone that the After-Hours Edge comes to life, a makeup look that embodies the mystique and allure of Manhattan's night. This is for the woman who navigates the transformation from boardroom powerhouse to evening sophisticate with effortless grace. Her eyeliner becomes more than a mere cosmetic; it's a tool of transformation, a symbol of her ability to blend the assertive energy of the day with the enigmatic charm of the night.

- **The Smoky Upgrade: Mysterious and Inviting**. Add depth to your daytime eyeliner with a smoky effect. Smudge the lines slightly and incorporate darker eyeshadow shades to create a look that's both mysterious and inviting, perfect for intimate gatherings or a post-work cocktail.
- **The Metallic Twist: Glamorous and Bold**. Introduce a hint of metallic eyeliner on top of your usual shade for a touch of glamour. This subtle addition catches the light and adds an extra dimension to your look, suitable for a night of dancing or a chic dinner party.
- **The Dramatic Lower Lash: Intensity and Intrigue**. Enhance the lower lash line with a more pronounced eyeliner application. This adds intensity to your gaze, perfect for those enigmatic encounters and deep conversations that fill Manhattan's after-hours scene.
- **The Bold Color Pop: Vibrant and Playful**. For a more adventurous look, add a pop of color with your eyeliner. Vibrant blues, greens, or purples can elevate your after-hours look, showcasing your playful side and adding a touch of whimsy to your evening escapades.

- **The Winged Evolution: From Sleek to Seductive**. Transform your daytime winged eyeliner into a more dramatic, elongated wing for the evening. This bolder wing adds an element of seduction and sophistication, perfect for capturing the essence of Manhattan's vibrant nightlife and making a statement in any upscale lounge or club.
- **The Inner Corner Highlight: Subtle Sparkle for Enigmatic Eyes**. Add a touch of shimmering highlight to the inner corners of your eyes. This subtle sparkle brings a playful yet sophisticated glow, illuminating your eyes and enhancing their allure, ideal for capturing attention in dimly lit settings.
- **The Layer Liner: Depth and Dimension**. Layer your eyeliner with different textures for added depth. A combination of gel, pencil, or liquid liner can create a multidimensional look that adds complexity and intrigue, mirroring the layered and multifaceted nature of Manhattan after dark.
- **Refined Glitter Line: Elegant Nighttime Sparkle**. Elevate your evening eyeliner by adding a thin line of refined glitter just above your traditional eyeliner. This delicate shimmer plays beautifully under low lights, enhancing the glamorous feel of your after-hours look without overwhelming, perfect for sophisticated night-outs where every detail is an understatement of elegance.

The After-Hours Edge is more than just a change in makeup; it's a celebration of the night's transformative power. It's a look that captures the essence of Manhattan after dark—a blend of mystery, allure, and sophistication. This eyeliner style is for the woman who thrives in the city's twilight, who embraces the night with open arms and a daring spirit. In this world where the skyline glitters and the streets whisper with untold stories, her eyes reflect the depth and dynamism of Manhattan's nocturnal beauty.

Completed Tasks: After-Hours Edge Activities

Inspirational Quote

NURTURE YOUR MINDS WITH GREAT THOUGHTS. TO BELIEVE IN THE HEROIC MAKES HEROES. — Benjamin Disraeli

Action Items: Intentions and Thoughts

The Maverick's Swoop

In the daring landscape of Manhattan, where innovation and boldness are the currencies of success, there emerges a look that's as audacious as the city itself—the Maverick's Swoop. This isn't just an eyeliner style; it's a declaration, a fearless expression of individuality and strength. For the woman who strides through the city carving her own path, who breaks conventions and sets trends, this eyeliner is her banner. The Maverick's Swoop is for the daring, for those who command the room not just with their ideas but with the sheer force of their presence. It's a style that speaks of risk-takers, of trailblazers, of those unafraid to make their mark in the bold script of Manhattan's ever-evolving story.

- **The Dramatic Wing: Defiance in a Stroke**. Embrace a wing that's more than just an extension—make it a dramatic, sweeping statement. This bold wing is a visual echo of the maverick's fearless approach to life and business, a symbol of her willingness to take risks and soar.

- **The Thick and Bold Line: Unapologetic and Commanding**. Opt for a thick, pronounced line that stands out unapologetically. This style is not about blending in; it's about standing out, about owning your space with confidence and undeniable presence.

- **The Edgy Accents: Innovative and Unconventional**. Incorporate unexpected accents into your eyeliner style, such as graphic lines or unusual color pops. These elements signify the maverick's creative and innovative spirit, showcasing her knack for thinking outside the box.

- **The Intense Color Palette: Vivid and Expressive**. Go beyond the traditional black or brown. Experiment with deep blues, greens, or even metallic hues to reflect the maverick's vibrant and unconventional approach to life and style.

- **The Dual-Toned Dynamism: Contrast and Character**. Experiment with dual-toned eyeliner, combining two contrasting shades for a dynamic and unique look. This style showcases the maverick's flair for combining diverse elements into a cohesive and striking statement, much like her approach to challenges and opportunities in Manhattan.
- **The Lower Lash Line Twist: Rebellious Underline**. Add an unexpected line along the lower lash line, perhaps even extending it parallel to the upper wing. This unconventional addition speaks to the maverick's rebellious nature, her readiness to flip the script and challenge traditional norms.
- **The Textured Technique: Bold and Artistic**. Play with textures by layering a matte eyeliner with a hint of glitter or gloss. This combination of textures reflects the multifaceted personality and her ability to blend pragmatism with a touch of the extraordinary.
- **The Futuristic Flick: Ahead of the Curve**. Incorporate futuristic elements into your eyeliner style, such as a sharply angled flick or geometric shapes. This forward-thinking approach to eyeliner mirrors the maverick's visionary outlook, always thinking ahead and setting trends rather than following them.

In the heart of Manhattan, where every street and skyscraper pulses with stories of ambition and success, the Maverick's Swoop stands as a testament to those who dare to be different. It's more than just an eyeliner style; it's an embodiment of the maverick spirit, a symbol of the courage to defy norms and the audacity to dream big. For the woman who wears it, it's not just a part of her makeup routine; it's a part of her identity, a bold stroke that mirrors her unique trajectory through the fast-paced, ever-changing world of Manhattan. In this city of endless possibilities, the Maverick's Swoop is not just a look; it's a statement of power, creativity, and unyielding individuality.

Completed Tasks: Maverick's Swoop Activities

Inspirational Quote

AS KNOWLEDGE INCREASES, WONDER DEEPENS. — Charles Morgan

Action Items: Intentions and Thoughts

Action Items: Intentions and Thoughts

Skyline Shadows: Eyeshadow Palettes that Mirror Manhattan's Horizon

Manhattan, where the skyline is more than just an array of buildings—it's a canvas, telling tales of aspirations that touch the clouds, desires that shimmer in twilight, and a boldness that turns day into dazzling night. Amidst this city of dreams, it's not just about witnessing the sunset or the dawn; it's about wearing them, each hue reflecting a chapter of New York's grand narrative.

Now, visualize this: You're gliding down Madison Avenue, and while the glint of your heels might capture a glance or two, it's the spectrum on your eyelids, mirroring the city's horizon, that's truly enchanting. That, darling, is the Skyline Shadow, an artistry that captures the essence of Manhattan, with every shade narrating stories of penthouses, parties, and dreams painted against the city's vast sky.

In this tantalizing chapter of The Manhattan Diaries, we dive into the world of eyeshadows, those sublime palettes that encapsulate the city's skyline—from the golden hues of dawn, the sultry tones of dusk, to the deep blues of a midnight escapade. Whether you wish for a subtle whisper of Central Park at day or the bold statement of Times Square in its nocturnal glory, you'll find your narrative here.

But it's more profound than just a sweep of color, It's an emotion, a sentiment, an ambition. It's about embodying Manhattan's panorama, celebrating both its towering achievements and the intimate, shadowed alleys where dreams take root.

So, join me on this journey, where we don't just witness the city's skyline, but wear it, embodying its tales and allure. Because, in Manhattan, every glance isn't just a fleeting moment—it's a saga. So, are you ready to paint your story? The palette of the city awaits. Dive into The Manhattan Diaries—where your gaze can capture the very soul of the cityscape.

Dawn's First Light

As Manhattan awakens to the first light of dawn, there's a rare tranquility in the air, a momentary pause in the city's relentless rhythm. It's during these early hours, as the first rays gently kiss the skyline, that Dawn's First Light in eyeshadow comes to life. This look captures the soft, serene beauty of the city at daybreak. It's for the woman who appreciates the quiet majesty of New York as it stirs from slumber, her makeup a reflection of the subtle yet striking colors that paint the sky. The palette is a harmony of soft pinks, gentle golds, and the lightest blues, reminiscent of the peaceful morning sky that overlooks the awakening city.

- **The Gentle Pink: Whisper of Daybreak**. Choose a soft pink eyeshadow, reminiscent of the delicate hues that appear in the sky as the city wakes. This color reflects the promise and hope of a new day, perfect for a fresh, understated look.
- **The Warm Gold: First Light's Embrace**. Incorporate warm gold tones to capture the essence of the first light. This shade mirrors the golden glow of sunrise, offering a hint of radiance and warmth to your look, symbolizing the city's slow illumination.
- **The Tranquil Blue: Sky's Soft Caress**. Add a touch of light blue to suggest the clear, tranquil morning sky. This color brings a sense of calm and serenity to your makeup, echoing the peaceful moments before the city bursts into life.
- **The Subtle Shimmer: Dewy Morning Glow**. Finish with a hint of shimmer to emulate the dewy freshness of dawn. A light application gives a natural, glowing effect, much like the dewdrops that glisten in the city's early light.
- **The Subdued Peach: The Blush of Awakening**. Integrate a soft peach shade into your palette to evoke the blush of the early morning

sun. This hue brings a touch of warmth and natural color, reminiscent of the subtle glow that bathes the city as it awakens.

- **The Whispering Lavender: Hints of Daybreak Dreams**. Add a hint of lavender to suggest the dreamy quality of dawn. This gentle color captures the ethereal nature of the early hours, reflecting the peaceful transition from night to day in the city.
- **The Creamy Matte: Soft Touch of Morning**. Use a creamy matte eyeshadow for a more natural, daybreak effect. This texture mimics the soft, muted quality of the morning light, perfect for creating a look that's understated yet impactful.
- **The Reflective Pearl: Glimmer of First Light**. Incorporate a touch of pearl or light ivory to highlight and brighten the eyes. This reflective shade captures the first gleaming light of daybreak, adding a subtle luminosity that mirrors the fresh start of a new day in Manhattan.
- **The Muted Taupe: Subtle City Silhouette**. Introduce a muted taupe shade to your palette to reflect the subtle contours of the cityscape at dawn. This earthy tone complements the lighter, airier colors, grounding the look with a hint of urban sophistication that echoes the quiet yet powerful awakening of Manhattan.

Dawn's First Light is more than just an eyeshadow style; it's a celebration of the calm and beauty of early morning in Manhattan. This look is for the woman who finds beauty in life's quiet moments, who sees the start of the day as a canvas of potential. Wearing this palette is like wearing a piece of the city's morning sky, a tribute to the gentle yet profound beauty of daybreak in New York. In a city that's always moving, this look captures the serene grace of its rare, peaceful moments.

Completed Tasks: Dawn's First Light Activities

Inspirational Quote

MEMORIES OF OUR LIVES, OF OUR WORKS, AND OTHER DEEDS WILL CONTINUE IN OTHERS. — Rosa Parks

Action Items: Intentions and Thoughts

Twilight's Sultry Spell

As the sun dips below the horizon, Manhattan cloaks itself in the enigmatic allure of twilight. This is when Twilight's Sultry Spell in eyeshadow captures the city's transition from the bustling energy of day to the mysterious charm of the evening. This look is for the woman who thrives in the city's dusky hours, her makeup a reflection of the deep, sultry tones that paint the sky. The palette is a mesmerizing blend of purples, deep blues, and smoky grays, reminiscent of the cityscape silhouetted against the evening sky. It's for those moments when the city's energy turns inward, becoming more intimate, more introspective.

- **The Deep Purple Haze: Mystery and Intrigue**. Embrace deep purple shades that evoke the mystery and intrigue of dusk. This color mirrors the rich hues of the twilight sky, perfect for creating an eyeshadow look that's both captivating and enigmatic.
- **The Smoky Blue: Evening's Embrace**. Incorporate smoky blue tones to reflect the transition from day to night. This shade represents the shadowy blue of the evening sky, adding a touch of sophistication and depth to your look, ideal for a night of exploration in Manhattan's vibrant nightlife.
- **The Seductive Gray: City's Nighttime Whisper**. Add elements of seductive gray to mimic the city's concrete bathed in the soft light of the moon and street lamps. It's a shade that speaks of the city's urban charm, creating an allure that's both modern and timeless.
- **The Shimmering Silver: Twilight's Sparkle**. A hint of shimmering silver can bring your twilight look to life. This touch captures the sparkle of the city's lights as they begin to twinkle against the night sky, adding a glimmer of excitement and anticipation for the night ahead.

- **The Midnight Navy: Depth of the Night Sky**. Introduce a shade of midnight navy to your eyeshadow palette. This deep, rich color embodies the vastness and depth of the night sky over Manhattan, perfect for adding a touch of sophisticated drama to your evening look.
- **The Glimmering Charcoal: Urban Glow**. Add a touch of glimmering charcoal to reflect the urban glow of the city streets. This smoky hue with subtle sparkles captures the essence of Manhattan's bustling nightlife, mirroring the shimmering lights of skyscrapers and bustling avenues.
- **The Rosy Dusk: Soft Twilight Blush**. Incorporate a hint of rosy dusk for a softer, more romantic aspect of twilight. This shade represents the fleeting moments of sunset, adding a warm, tender glow to your twilight makeup, perfect for an evening of romance or a sophisticated dinner.
- **The Metallic Bronze: Reflections of Sunset**. A touch of metallic bronze can add warmth and richness to your twilight look. This shade evokes the last golden rays of the setting sun reflecting off Manhattan's buildings, bringing a final hint of day's warmth to the cool palette of the evening.

Twilight's Sultry Spell is more than just an eyeshadow style; it's a homage to the transformative power of evening in Manhattan. This look is for the woman who commands the night, who finds her energy in the city's twilight hours. Wearing this palette is like wearing a piece of Manhattan's night sky, a tribute to the moments when the city transitions from the clarity of day to the mystery of night. In a place where every evening holds the promise of a new adventure, this look captures the allure and depth of Manhattan as it embraces the night.

Completed Tasks: Twilight's Sultry Spell Activities

Inspirational Quote

CHERISH YOUR VISIONS AND YOUR DREAMS AS THEY ARE THE CHILDREN OF YOUR SOUL, THE BLUEPRINTS OF YOUR ULTIMATE ACHIEVEMENTS. —Napoleon Hill

Action Items: Intentions and Thoughts

Midnight's Majesty

In Manhattan, the stroke of midnight ushers in a realm where glamour and mystery reign supreme. This is the domain of Midnight's Majesty, an eyeshadow palette as enigmatic as the city itself. For the nocturnal beauties who revel under starlit skies, these shades—from electric blue to shimmering silver—capture the essence of Manhattan's vibrant nightlife. Each color tells a story of midnight escapades and whispered secrets, perfect for the woman who commands the dark with elegance and allure. Dive into the majestic spirit of the city that never sleeps, and let your eyes do all the talking.

- **The Energy of the Night: Midnight's Majesty**. Immerse yourself in the intensity of electric blue eyeshadow. This shade captures the dynamic energy of Manhattan's nightlife, perfect for a bold look that resonates with the vibrancy of late-night city escapades.

- **The Shimmering Silver: City Lights Aglow**. Incorporate shimmering silver to reflect the glittering lights of the city. This shade adds a touch of glamour and sophistication, mirroring the sparkle of Manhattan's skyline as it lights up the night.

- **The Dramatic Black: Mystery of the Metropolis**. Embrace the depth and mystery of the night with a dramatic black eyeshadow. This color embodies the enigmatic allure of Manhattan after dark, perfect for a seductive, powerful look that commands attention.

- **The Starlit Shimmer: Twinkle of the Night Sky**. Add a hint of starlit shimmer to your eyeshadow. This subtle sparkle brings a magical quality to your look, reminiscent of the stars twinkling above the city's soaring skyscrapers.

- **The Cosmic Cobalt: Depth of the Night Sky**. Integrate a deep cobalt shade to mirror the rich, velvety depth of the night sky. This bold and sophisticated hue adds a sense of majesty and mystery, ideal for capturing the essence of a starry Manhattan night.

- **The Gleaming Gunmetal: Sleek and Modern**. Add a touch of gleaming gunmetal to your palette. This modern, metallic shade reflects the sleek and sophisticated side of Manhattan's nightlife, perfect for a look that's both edgy and elegant.
- **The Intense Plum: Sultry and Enigmatic**. Incorporate a deep plum shade to bring warmth and intensity to your midnight palette. This rich, enigmatic color is reminiscent of the hidden gems and secret rendezvous spots scattered throughout the city after dark.
- **The Iridescent Moonlight: Soft and Ethereal**. Use a hint of iridescent moonlight shade to add a soft, ethereal touch to your look. This light, shimmering color captures the gentle glow of the moon over the city, providing a subtle contrast to the darker, more dramatic shades.
- **The Velvet Violet: Rich and Romantic**. Add a touch of velvet violet to your eyeshadow palette for a rich, romantic finish. This luxurious shade brings a layer of depth and passion to your look, ideal for those moments when the city's midnight charm calls for a hint of mysterious elegance.

Midnight's Majesty is not just an eyeshadow style; it's a celebration of Manhattan's nocturnal wonder. It's for the woman who finds magic in the city's after-hours, who is captivated by the mystery and allure of the night. Wearing this palette is like wearing a piece of the city's nightscape, a tribute to the allure and mystique that Manhattan exudes under the cover of darkness. In a city where the night is as alive as the day, this look captures the essence of its majestic, vibrant spirit, perfect for those who embrace the night and all its endless possibilities.

Completed Tasks: Midnight's Majesty Activities

Inspirational Quote

IT IS ONLY IN SORROW BAD WEATHER MATTERS TO US; IN JOY WE FACE THE STORM AND DEFY IT. — Amelia Barr

Action Items: Intentions and Thoughts

The Urban Spectrum

In the ever-changing landscape of Manhattan, where every corner boasts a different hue and every moment a different mood, the Urban Spectrum of eyeshadows captures the essence of the city in its entirety. This is for the woman who seeks to embody the full range of Manhattan's diverse character, from the fresh serenity of Central Park mornings to the electric buzz of Times Square at midnight. The Urban Spectrum palette is a celebration of the city's dynamic beauty, offering a versatile collection of colors that can adapt to any setting, any time, any mood. It's a tribute to the multifaceted spirit of New York, where diversity is not just embraced but celebrated.

- **The Morning Neutrals: Soft and Subtle for Daylight Hours**. Begin with a range of neutral shades for the daytime. Soft beiges, light browns, and gentle pinks mirror the calm and hopeful energy of Manhattan mornings, perfect for a day at the office or a casual brunch in the Upper West Side.
- **The Afternoon Pastels: Colorful and Playful for Sunny Afternoons**. As the day progresses, introduce pastel shades into your look. Light blues, greens, and lavenders capture the playful spirit of a sunny afternoon in Manhattan, ideal for a stroll through SoHo or a visit to one of the city's many museums.
- **The Evening Riches: Deep and Luxurious for Nightfall**. For the evening, transition to richer, deeper shades. Dark purples, blues, and emerald greens reflect the luxurious and mysterious vibe of Manhattan's nightlife, suited for an elegant dinner in the Meatpacking District or a Broadway show.
- **The Sunset Oranges: Warm and Radiant for Evening Transition**. As the day gives way to evening, embrace warm orange and coral shades. These colors capture the stunning beauty of a Manhattan sunset, perfect for a transition look that's both radiant

and inviting, ideal for an early evening cocktail or a walk along the Hudson River.

- **The Metallic Bronzes: Sophisticated and Earthy for Any Occasion**. Incorporate metallic bronze tones for a sophisticated yet earthy effect. This versatile shade can add depth to both day and night looks, resonating with the city's blend of natural elements and urban sophistication, suitable for any occasion in Manhattan's diverse social landscape.
- **The Classic Blacks and Grays: Sleek and Timeless for Enduring Elegance**. Include classic blacks and grays for creating sleek, timeless looks. These shades are essential for achieving the quintessential New York style, embodying the city's enduring elegance and its iconic, ever-present skyline.
- **The Nighttime Glitters: Bold and Bright for the City That Never Sleeps**. Finally, the palette offers bold, glittering shades for the late-night hours. Think shimmering golds, silvers, and metallics that capture the vibrant energy of Times Square at night, perfect for a club in Chelsea or a late-night rooftop party.

The Urban Spectrum is more than just a collection of eyeshadows; it's an ode to the vibrancy and diversity of Manhattan. Each shade is a reflection of the city's myriad faces, from the gentle light of dawn to the bold colors of the night. For the woman who wears this palette, each color is a chance to explore a different side of herself, just as she explores the many sides of the city. In Manhattan, where change is the only constant, the Urban Spectrum palette is her companion through every transformation, every adventure, every moment.

Completed Tasks: Urban Spectrum Activities

Inspirational Quote

SHOOT FOR THE MOON AND IF YOU MISS, YOU WILL STILL BE AMONG THE STARS. — Les Brown

Action Items: Intentions and Thoughts

Action Items: Intentions and Thoughts

Fifth Avenue Flutter: Lashes that Speak Volumes

Manhattan, a city that whispers tales of grandeur at every corner, where every fluttering curtain and flag echoes ambition, desire, and a drama worthy of Broadway's limelight. In this metropolis of ceaseless momentum, it's not just about charting your path; it's about marking it—with a splash of elegance, a flair of sophistication, and a look that's simply unforgettable.

Imagine this scenario: You're sauntering down Fifth Avenue, the rhythm of your heels syncing with the heartbeat of the city. Every gaze that meets yours isn't just captivated by the sway of your silhouette, but by the mesmerizing dance of your lashes. That, my dear, is the Fifth Avenue Flutter, an ocular symphony that whispers tales of nights at the opera, candlelit dinners, and secret rendezvous.

In this enticing chapter of The Manhattan Diaries, you'll delve into the world of lashes that aren't just long, but tell long tales. From the subtle allure of a morning brunch to the dramatic flair of a midnight gala, you'll uncover the art of selecting and flaunting lashes that can stop the city in its tracks.

But there's more to it than meets the eye. It's about wearing a sentiment, an emotion, an entire narrative on those delicate fringes. It's about reflecting Manhattan's elegance, its pulse, its undying charm, and the myriad tales that lie in its shadows and bright lights.

So, accompany me as we navigate through the serenades sung from the quaint cafes to the dazzling ballrooms, enhancing the art of a gaze that doesn't just attract, but resonates with stories and dreams. Because, darling, in Manhattan, every blink is an opportunity, a statement, a story waiting to be told. Are you ready for your close-up? The city's spotlight awaits. Dive into The Manhattan Diaries—where your eyes become the windows to Manhattan's soul.

The Brunch Bash Lash

In the light and airy atmosphere of a Manhattan morning, where the city basks in the soft glow of the sun and the clink of brunch glasses fills the air, there emerges a beauty essential—the Brunch Bash Lash. This lash style is for the woman who graces the chicest brunch spots on Fifth Avenue, her presence as effortless as it is elegant. The Brunch Bash Lash is not about overt drama; it's about enhancing natural beauty with a touch of sophistication, perfect for those leisurely mornings spent under the open skies of rooftop cafes or in the quaint corners of a park-side bistro.

- **The Soft Flutter: Understated Charm**. Opt for lashes that offer a soft flutter, enhancing your eyes with a natural yet polished look. This style is perfect for adding a hint of refinement without appearing overdone, embodying the relaxed yet chic vibe of a Manhattan brunch.
- **The Light Volume: Subtle Fullness**. Choose lashes that provide a light volume, giving your eyes a bright, open appearance. This subtle fullness is ideal for morning gatherings, striking the right balance between casual charm and understated glamour.
- **The Delicate Length: Elongated Elegance**. Select lashes that offer a delicate lengthening effect. This adds a touch of elegance, elongating the eyes gracefully, perfect for a day of leisure and conversation in the city's sunlit venues.
- **The Natural Curve: Soft and Approachable**. Embrace lashes with a gentle curve that mimic your natural lash line. This approachable style complements the daytime's soft light and the laid-back ambiance of a New York brunch.
- **The Feathery Touch: Light and Airy**. Choose lashes that have a feathery, lightweight quality. This style adds a breezy, carefree

elegance to your look, mirroring the relaxed yet sophisticated atmosphere of a Manhattan brunch on a sunlit terrace.

- **The Subtle Accent: Enhancing Natural Beauty**. Incorporate lashes that accentuate rather than transform. This style is about enhancing your natural lashes with a subtle boost, ideal for a look that's both authentic and refined, suitable for a casual catch-up with friends or a leisurely morning read.
- **The Tapered Finish: Softly Defined Edges**. Opt for lashes that taper at the ends, providing a soft, natural finish. This delicate tapering gives a gentle lift to the eyes, perfect for creating a look that's inviting and open, in tune with the friendly and laid-back vibe of brunch gatherings.
- **The Minimalist Approach: Less Is More**. Embrace a minimalist approach with lashes that offer just enough enhancement to make a difference, yet maintain a natural look. This style is all about understatement, echoing the effortless chic that's synonymous with Manhattan's brunch scene.

The Brunch Bash Lash is the quintessential choice for the Manhattanite who revels in the city's morning allure. It's a celebration of the casual elegance that defines New York's brunch culture, where beauty is effortless and style is innate. These lashes don't just enhance a look; they capture the essence of a relaxed yet sophisticated morning, making every blink an expression of understated grace. In the world of The Manhattan Diaries, where brunch is an event and style is paramount, the Brunch Bash Lash is your secret to mastering the art of daytime elegance.

Completed Tasks: Brunch Bash Lash Activities

Inspirational Quote

ACCEPT THE THINGS TO WHICH FATE BINDS YOU AND LOVE THE PEOPLE WITH WHOM FATE BRINGS YOU TOGETHER—BUT DO SO WITH ALL YOUR HEART. — Marcus Aurelius

Action Items: Intentions and Thoughts

The Boardroom Bold

In the high-stakes environment of Manhattan's boardrooms, where decisions shape destinies and confidence is key, emerges a lash style that speaks volumes—the Boardroom Bold. This look is for the woman who commands attention not just with her ideas but with her presence, a presence accentuated by lashes that are as bold and assertive as her business acumen. The Boardroom Bold lashes are not about blending in; they're about standing out, embodying the strength and determination required to thrive in the corporate jungle of New York. They're for the woman who strides into meetings with the assurance that she's not just part of the conversation; she's leading it.

- **The Defined Volume: Impactful Presence**. Choose lashes that provide a defined volume, making a statement without overshadowing your professional demeanor. This style conveys confidence and power, essential for holding sway in the boardroom.
- **The Structured Length: Commanding Yet Refined**. Opt for lashes with a noticeable length that maintains a refined shape. This structured look mirrors the precision and control needed in corporate decision-making, perfect for exuding authority and sophistication.
- **The Dramatic Curl: Bold and Captivating**. Embrace a dramatic curl in your lashes to draw focus to your eyes, ensuring that when you speak, all eyes are on you. This bold curl is about making every glance impactful, a reflection of your bold ideas and dynamic leadership.
- **The Intense Thickness: Unyielding Determination**. Select lashes that offer an intense thickness, symbolizing the unyielding determination and resilience required in the business world. This

look is assertive and unapologetic, much like the attitude needed to navigate the complexities of corporate Manhattan.

- **The Sleek Separation: Precision and Poise**. Focus on lashes that offer sleek separation, avoiding clumps for a polished and professional appearance. This style reflects precision and poise, mirroring the clarity and focus required in high-level business discussions and negotiations.
- **The Natural Hue: Subtle Yet Strong**. While embracing boldness, opt for lashes in natural hues like deep browns or blacks. These shades are powerful yet understated, ensuring your look remains authoritative without appearing overly dramatic, suitable for the professional decorum of the boardroom.
- **The Fuller Outer Edge: Strategic Emphasis**. Consider lashes that are fuller at the outer edge, creating a subtle cat-eye effect. This design subtly enhances the eye's shape, conveying strategic insight and a forward-thinking mindset, key attributes in the corporate world.
- **The Balanced Impact: Confident and Composed**. Aim for a balance between impact and elegance. Lashes should be bold enough to make a statement but not so overpowering that they detract from your overall presence.

The Boardroom Bold lashes are more than just a beauty choice; they're a tool of empowerment in the corporate world. For the Manhattan woman who knows her worth and isn't afraid to show it, these lashes are a badge of her ambition and her capability. In the city where business is as much about perception as it is about performance, the Boardroom Bold lashes are her allies, accentuating not just her eyes but her entire persona. In a place where the stakes are high and the competition fierce, these lashes ensure she not only participates but dominates, making every blink.

Completed Tasks: Boardroom Bold Activities

Inspirational Quote

WE HAVE IT IN OUR POWER TO BEGIN THE WORLD OVER AGAIN. — Thomas Paine

Action Items: Intentions and Thoughts

The Evening Elegance

As the sun sets over the Manhattan skyline, the city transitions into an enchanting world of evening elegance. In these magical twilight hours, the Evening Elegance lash style comes into play, perfect for the woman who graces the city's most exclusive soirees and nightspots. This lash look is about sophistication and allure, a perfect blend of drama and refinement. It's for the woman who commands the night with her charm and style, her lashes fluttering like the feathers of a mysterious, nocturnal bird. The Evening Elegance is not just a makeup choice; it's a statement of the night, embodying the glamour and sophistication that come alive in Manhattan as the day turns to night.

- **The Luxurious Length: Graceful and Refined**. Opt for lashes that offer luxurious length, extending your natural lash line with elegance and grace. This style enhances your eyes' natural beauty, perfect for a sophisticated night at the opera or a high-end gala event.
- **The Voluminous Curl: Captivating and Bold**. Embrace lashes with a voluminous curl, adding an element of boldness to your evening look. This curl lifts the eyes, making them more captivating and expressive, ideal for engaging in deep conversations at an intimate dinner party or while attending a Broadway premiere.
- **The Subtle Drama: Understated Yet Impactful**. Choose lashes that provide a subtle hint of drama without being over the top. This style is about adding depth and intensity to your look in a refined manner, mirroring the understated elegance of Manhattan's elite evening events.
- **The Delicate Density: Full and Feathered**. Select lashes that offer delicate density, creating a full and feathered effect. This look adds a

touch of glamour to your eyes, perfect for a night of dancing at an exclusive club or a romantic evening stroll along the Hudson River.

- **The Glittering Accent: Sparkle and Shine**. Introduce a touch of glitter or subtle shimmer on the tips of the lashes. This hint of sparkle catches the light beautifully, echoing the twinkling lights of Manhattan's skyline at night, perfect for adding a magical touch to your evening look.
- **The Winged Wonder: Sweeping and Sophisticated**. Consider lashes that gently wing out at the corners. This sweeping effect gracefully extends the eye, adding a hint of classic, sophisticated drama suitable for a grand entrance at a high-profile event or an elegant night at an upscale lounge.
- **Tapered Elegance: Natural to Bold Gradation**. Choose lashes that taper from natural at the inner corner to bold at the outer edge. This gradation in intensity creates a captivating look that's both natural and striking, embodying the seamless transition from the elegant simplicity of early evening to the vibrant energy of late-night Manhattan.

The Evening Elegance lash style is the quintessential expression of Manhattan's night-time allure. For the woman who adorns herself with these lashes, every blink is a moment of enchantment, every glance a spell of sophistication. In the city that shines brightest under the moonlight, these lashes are not just an accessory; they're a reflection of the night itself-mysterious, captivating, and irresistibly elegant. In the world of The Manhattan Diaries, where evenings are as enchanting as the cityscape itself, the Evening Elegance is your key to unlocking the magic of Manhattan nights.

Completed Tasks: Evening Elegance Activities

Inspirational Quote

IF YOU ACCEPT THE EXPECTATIONS OF OTHERS, ESPECIALLY NEGATIVE ONES, THEN YOU NEVER WILL CHANGE THE OUTCOME. — Michael Jordan

Action Items: Intentions and Thoughts

The Gala Glitz

In the opulent ballrooms and grand halls of Manhattan, where the elite gather under chandeliers and the air sparkles with sophistication, emerges the Gala Glitz lash style. This is the realm of high society, where every detail is a stroke of artistry, and every glance holds a story of luxury and allure. The Gala Glitz is for the woman who is not just attending the gala; she is part of its spectacle. Her lashes are a crowning touch to her ensemble, as bold and captivating as the city's most extravagant soirees. In this world of unapologetic glamour and elegance, her lashes are her most expressive accessory, speaking volumes of her presence and the magnetic charm she exudes.

- **The Dramatic Volume: Bold and Unforgettable**. Embrace lashes that boast dramatic volume, making a bold statement that's befitting the grandeur of a gala event. These lashes are all about presence, ensuring.
- **The Luxurious Length: Sophistication in Every Flutter**. Opt for lashes that extend with luxurious length, offering a sophisticated flutter that's perfect for a night of opulence. This style adds an element of high-class elegance, enhancing your eyes with the allure and mystery fitting for a Manhattan gala.
- **The Intense Curl: Captivating and Commanding**. Choose lashes with an intense curl that lifts and opens the eyes dramatically. This curl not only elevates your look but also commands attention, mirroring the grandeur and prestige of the gala scene.
- **The Shimmering Embellishment: Glimmering with Elegance**. Incorporate lashes with subtle shimmer or embellishments. This touch of sparkle reflects the glittering lights of the gala, adding a hint of enchanting glamour to your overall look, perfect for a night where every detail shines.

- **The Feathered Flair: Graceful and Flowing**. Add a dimension of grace with feathered lashes that flow seamlessly. This style imparts a sense of elegance and softness, evoking the luxurious gowns and flowing fabrics often seen at gala events, perfect for adding a touch of refined sophistication to your look.
- **The Bold Corner Highlight: Dramatic and Focused**. Consider lashes that are bolder and more voluminous at the outer corners. This focused drama draws attention to your eyes, mimicking the dramatic flair of a grand entrance, ideal for capturing the essence of the gala's theatricality.
- **Multi-Layered Luxe: Depth and Complexity**. Choose lashes that offer a multi-layered effect, adding depth and complexity. This style reflects the multifaceted nature of a gala event, where layers of luxury and opulence come together, perfect for a look that's as intricate and captivating as the evening itself.
- **The Sculpted Silhouette: Architecturally Inspired**. Opt for lashes that have a sculpted, architectural design, mimicking the structured lines and bold contours of Manhattan's skyline. This unique shape not only enhances the eye's natural beauty but also adds a modern twist to classic glamour, making it a standout choice.

The Gala Glitz lash style is more than just a beauty choice; it's an embodiment of the grandeur and magnificence of Manhattan's gala scene. For the woman who adorns herself with these lashes, every blink is a display of elegance, every gaze a testament to her allure. In a city where extravagance and sophistication go hand in hand, these lashes are not just an accessory; they are a declaration of her stature and style. In the world of The Manhattan Diaries, where galas are the ultimate showcase of splendor, the Gala Glitz lashes are your key to unlocking the allure of Manhattan's most enchanting nights.

Completed Tasks: Gala Glitz Activities

Inspirational Quote

IT IS IN YOUR MOMENTS OF DECISION THAT YOUR DESTINY IS SHAPED. — Tony Robbins

Action Items: Intentions and Thoughts

Action Items: Intentions and Thoughts

The Greenwich Glow: Highlighters and Bronzers for That Gilded Finish

Manhattan, a city of dreams and silhouettes, where every ray of sunlight bouncing off its iconic structures narrates tales of dreams realized, passions pursued, and the golden opportunities seized by its daring denizens. In this maze of ambition and elegance, it isn't simply about leaving a mark; it's about gleaming, glowing, and making sure that mark is gilded.

Picture this: You're sweeping through the historic pathways of Greenwich Village, and as the golden hour caresses the city, it captures the ethereal luminescence on your cheeks. It isn't the sequins on your attire, nor the diamonds on your fingers. Instead, it's the Greenwich Glow, an epitome of opulence, a hint of sun-kissed allure and moonlit mystique.

In this shimmering chapter of The Manhattan Diaries, we'll dive deep into the world of highlighters and bronzers that don't just add a glow, but tell a story. From the delicate radiance of a Sunday brunch to the robust bronzed aura of a rooftop soiree, discover the art of wearing the city's golden hours on your skin.

But hold on, it's not just about painting your face. It's about embodying the city's golden legacy, its highs and lows, its dawn and dusk. It's about wearing the stories of old townhouses, jazz bars, art alleys, and the ever-changing skyline, all in one stroke.

So, come with me, as we waltz through tree-lined streets, past historic brownstones, drawing inspiration from the city's ever-present glow, mastering the art of a finish that not only complements your stride but mirrors the city's gilded tales. Because, darling, in Manhattan, every gleam is a glimpse into the epic saga. Get ready, for the city is your canvas. Step into The Manhattan Diaries—where your glow is as timeless as the tales of the city itself.

The Brunch Radiance

In Manhattan, where brunch is a glamorous social event, a woman's glow is her finest accessory. Imagine stepping into a trendy Upper East Side eatery, radiating like a Manhattan sunrise. This is Brunch Radiance, an aura of leisure and luxury. In this chapter of The Manhattan Diaries, we explore how to achieve that envied glow. From elite skincare rituals to transformative makeup techniques, discover how to perfect a flawless radiance that speaks volumes, effortlessly.

- **Morning Rituals of Manhattan's Elite**. Delve into the morning skincare routines of Manhattan's upper echelon, discovering the luxurious products and techniques that keep their skin looking fresh and radiant. Start your day with a pampering routine that sets the tone for brunch with confidence.

- **The Luminous Canvas**. Explore makeup tips and tricks that allow you to create a luminous canvas for your brunch look. From foundation choices that mimic the perfection of a Manhattan townhouse facade to highlighting techniques that catch the light like skyscraper windows, discover how to achieve a radiant complexion that lasts through brunch and beyond.

- **The Effortless Glow**. Uncover the secrets of achieving a natural, effortless radiance that complements your brunch attire. From soft, dewy lips that evoke the sweetness of pastries to a subtle smoky eye that mirrors the city's smoldering skyline, embrace makeup techniques that enhance your features without overwhelming your brunch look.

- **The Confidence of Brunch Radiance**. Embrace the confidence that comes with your Brunch Radiance. Understand how looking and feeling your best can elevate your presence in Manhattan's elite social circles, much like a well-timed brunch reservation at the city's hottest spot. Step into the brunch scene with a glow that speaks of success, sophistication, and the allure of a Manhattan morning.

- **From Central Park Glow to Tribeca Tint**. Explore the neighborhood-inspired brunch radiance styles that Manhattan's fashionistas are currently embracing. Whether it's the natural, sun-kissed glow of Central Park or the edgy, downtown vibe of Tribeca, learn how to adapt your brunch radiance to match your chosen brunch locale.
- **Signature Scents for Brunch**. Discover the art of choosing the perfect fragrance for your brunch outings. Manhattan's elite understand the impact of a signature scent, and you'll learn how to select fragrances that complement your radiant brunch look and leave a lasting impression.
- **Brunch Radiance Beyond Brunch**. Understand how to maintain your brunch radiance throughout the day, whether you're attending meetings, exploring the city, or enjoying an afternoon at the museum. Your glow should endure like a Manhattan sunset, casting a warm and captivating light on everything you do.
- **The Art of Layering**. Master the art of layering skincare and makeup products to achieve a multidimensional glow. Combine serums, moisturizers, and primers that not only enhance your skin's natural radiance but also ensure your makeup stays flawless throughout your brunch and beyond. This skill is key to a luminous appearance that captures and reflects a Manhattan morning.

As you sip your latte and savor your eggs benedict, remember that in Manhattan, brunch isn't just a meal; it's a lifestyle. Your Brunch Radiance is your passport to this exclusive world of indulgence, and it's time to shine. Welcome to The Manhattan Diaries, where your radiant presence at brunch is your best-kept secret.

Completed Tasks: Brunch Radiance Activities

Inspirational Quote

EVERYTHING YOU WANT IS OUT THERE WAITING FOR YOU TO ASK. EVERYTHING YOU WANT ALSO WANTS YOU. BUT YOU HAVE TO TAKE ACTION TO GET IT. — Jules Renard

Action Items: Intentions and Thoughts

The Afternoon Allure

Manhattan, a city where time seems to slow down in the golden hours of the afternoon, offering a brief respite from the hustle of the day. It's during this magical time that the city's elite gather to bask in the warm glow of success, style, and sophistication. In the heart of Manhattan's chicest spots, afternoon allure takes center stage, and the city's most glamorous residents know how to make the most of it. Join me on this enchanting journey as we unlock the secrets to mastering the art of the Afternoon Allure, a chapter in The Manhattan Diaries that will elevate your daytime elegance to new heights.

- **The Afternoon Allure Essentials**. To create an irresistible afternoon allure, you'll need the right tools. Dive into skincare routines that leave your complexion radiant and explore makeup techniques that accentuate your best features, ensuring you're ready to shine.

- **Manhattan's Afternoon Hideaways**. Manhattan is a treasure trove of hidden gems, from charming tea rooms to rooftop lounges. Discover the perfect settings for showcasing your afternoon allure and learn how to match your ambiance to your allure.

- **Wardrobe Wizardry**. Your choice of attire plays a pivotal role in your afternoon allure. Whether it's a flowing summer dress or a tailored ensemble, explore how to select the ideal wardrobe pieces that enhance your allure and make you the star of the afternoon.

- **Accessories That Dazzle**. Accessories can elevate your look to the next level. From statement jewelry to elegant handbags, we'll guide you in choosing pieces that complement your style and draw admiration wherever you go.

- **Afternoon Allure Conversations**. Engaging in captivating conversations is a hallmark of Manhattan's elite. Discover the art of witty banter and engaging dialogue that will leave a memorable impression during your social encounters.

- **The Power of Poise**. Poise and posture are essential for exuding afternoon allure. Explore the nuances of body language, grace, and confidence to leave a lasting impression wherever you venture.
- **Capturing Your Afternoon Allure**. Learn how to document and preserve your moments of afternoon allure through photography. Take perfect selfies, candid shots, or professionally captured photos that showcase your radiant self.
- **Afternoon Allure Beyond Manhattan**. Extend your newfound allure beyond the city's borders. Whether you're on a weekend getaway, vacation, or business trip, explore how to maintain your captivating presence, ensuring that your allure knows no geographical limits.
- **Afternoon Allure Legacy**. Discover the art of leaving a legacy of afternoon allure. Your charisma and elegance can inspire others and create a lasting impact, not only in Manhattan but in the hearts of those you encounter.
- **Unveiling Your Inner Siren**. In the grand finale, we'll guide you in tapping into your inner siren, allowing you to unleash your full potential. By the end of this chapter, you'll possess the knowledge and confidence to effortlessly exude afternoon allure and leave an indelible mark on Manhattan's social scene.

As the sun gently fades behind Manhattan's skyline, remember that every moment in this city holds the promise of enchantment. The Afternoon Allure offers you the chance to shine your brightest. In Manhattan, your allure is your secret weapon, turning every moment into magic.

Completed Tasks: Afternoon Allure Activities

Inspirational Quote

PLANT THY FOOT FIRMLY IN THE PRINTS WHICH HIS FOOT HAS MADE BEFORE THEE. — Joseph Barber Lightfoot

Action Items: Intentions and Thoughts

The Twilight Shimmer

As twilight blankets the city that never sleeps, Manhattan undergoes a breathtaking transformation. The bustling streets take on a softer glow, the city's energy evolves into something more intimate, and every corner seems to whisper secrets of the night ahead. It's during this enchanting hour that you step into the limelight, with a shimmer that captures the essence of Manhattan's nocturnal allure.

- **The Twilight Shimmer Palette**. Allow yourself to be swept away by the curated collection of shades that define the Twilight Shimmer look. From the ethereal champagne highlights that mimic the city's glistening skyscrapers to the smoky grays that evoke the mysterious allure of Manhattan's cobblestone streets, these shades are your passport to the city's twilight secrets.
- **Creating a Subtle Canvas**. Before you embark on your journey into the world of Twilight Shimmer, discover the art of achieving a flawless base. Your skin is the canvas, and proper skincare and foundation are your tools. Prepare to unveil a complexion that's as smooth and inviting as a moonlit river.
- **Eyes that Mesmerize**. Dive into the techniques that make your eyes the focal point of the Twilight Shimmer. With a step-by-step guide, master the art of achieving the perfect smoky eye. These sultry, smoldering eyes are the windows to your Manhattan twilight adventures.
- **Cheeks Aglow**. Capture the romantic essence of the Manhattan twilight with cheeks that radiate a soft, rosy glow. Your blush is the brushstroke that adds warmth and charm to your canvas, mirroring the city's romantic ambiance as night falls.

- **The Lips Speak Volumes**. The final touch in your transformation into a Manhattan twilight goddess is your lip shade. Learn how to select the ideal hue that complements your Twilight Shimmer. Whether it's a subtle nude that Whispers secrets or a bold red that commands attention, your lips will convey the unspoken stories of your night.
- **The Enigmatic Perfume**. Just as Manhattan transforms during twilight, your scent should be equally captivating. Explore the fragrances that evoke the essence of the city after dark. From seductive notes of amber and musk to the allure of floral bouquets, choose a perfume that leaves a trail of intrigue in your wake.
- **Accessories for the Night**. Enhance your Twilight Shimmer with carefully selected accessories that reflect the city's mystique. Delve into the world of jewelry, from delicate pieces that twinkle like starlight to bold statement pieces that command attention. Each accessory tells a tale of elegance and allure.
- **The Manhattan Twilight Wardrobe**. Complement your makeup with a wardrobe that mirrors Manhattan's twilight magic. Discover the fabrics and styles that capture the city's essence. From flowing silks that mimic the play of city lights on the river to tailored suits that exude sophistication, your attire should be an extension of your twilight persona.

As dusk descends, your Twilight Shimmer look becomes your passport to Manhattan's enchanted evening scene. Each brushstroke and accessory choice crafts a narrative of glamour and mystery, perfectly echoing the city's sparkling twilight. Step out and let your shimmer blend with the city's glow, making every moment a captivating chapter in Manhattan's nightlife. Tonight, the city is unmistakably yours.

Completed Tasks: Twilight Shimmer Activities

Inspirational Quote

EVERYTHING YOU WANT IS OUT THERE WAITING FOR YOU TO ASK. EVERYTHING YOU WANT ALSO WANTS YOU. BUT YOU HAVE TO TAKE ACTION TO GET IT. — Miya Yamanouchi

Action Items: Intentions and Thoughts

The Nighttime Glamour

In the city that never sleeps, the night is a stage, and your presence should be nothing short of spectacular. Whether you're sipping cocktails in a hidden speakeasy or attending a glamorous gala, Manhattan's nightlife demands a level of allure that matches its dazzling streets. This chapter of The Manhattan Diaries delves into the art of Nighttime Glamour, where every detail of your look is a nod to the city's enchanting after-hours atmosphere.

- **Lustrous Nighttime Makeup**. When the sun sets, it's your time to shine. Embrace sultry, smoky eyes that capture the essence of a city bathed in twilight. Explore the world of shimmery eyeshadows, long-lasting mascaras, and bold eyeliners that create an enigmatic gaze. Your makeup should be a symphony of seduction, drawing admirers into your mysterious allure.

- **The Power of Lipstick**. In Manhattan's nightlife, your lips should do the talking. Discover the spectrum of lip colors that can transform your look from elegant to daring. From classic reds that exude confidence to deep plum shades that hint at intrigue, your choice of lipstick becomes a statement of intent.

- **The Allure of Hairstyling**. Your hair should be an extension of your Nighttime Glamour. Consider the sleek sophistication of an updo, the romantic allure of loose waves, or the bold statement of a faux hawk. Your hairstyle sets the mood for the evening, complementing your overall aura of enchantment.

- **Captivating Fragrances**. As the night unfolds, leave a trail of mesmerizing scents that linger in the memory. Explore fragrances that evoke the magic of Manhattan's nocturnal landscape. Whether it's the deep, woody notes of oud or the floral sweetness of jasmine, your choice of perfume should be a secret weapon in your arsenal of allure.

- **Statement Accessories**. Nighttime Glamour calls for accessories that leave a lasting impression. Explore the world of bold necklaces, statement earrings, and intricately designed bracelets that elevate your ensemble. These pieces should be conversation starters, adding depth and dimension to your overall look.
- **The Perfect LBD**. The Little Black Dress is a timeless canvas for Nighttime Glamour. Invest in a classic LBD that fits you like a dream and can be dressed up or down with the right accessories. It's your go-to choice for impromptu soirees and elegant gatherings.
- **Effortless Confidence**. Perhaps the most crucial element of Nighttime Glamour is confidence. It's not just about what you wear; it's about how you wear it. Carry yourself with an air of self-assuredness, knowing that you're a captivating presence in the city's glittering nightlife. Your confidence is the final touch that completes your Nighttime Glamour ensemble, making you unforgettable in Manhattan's star-studded evenings.
- **Chic Footwear Choices**. Elevate your Nighttime Glamour with the perfect pair of shoes. Whether it's stiletto heels that add a touch of sophistication or sleek ankle boots that merge comfort with style, your footwear should be as statement-making as your ensemble. Choose shoes that not only complement your outfit but also let you navigate Manhattan's nightlife with ease and poise.

In the heart of Manhattan's nightlife, your transformation into a beacon of Nighttime Glamour is not just a beauty ritual; it's an art form. Each element of your look, from makeup to hairstyle to fragrance, should resonate with the city's electrifying energy. As you step into the night, remember that Manhattan's streets are your runway, and the world is your audience. In The Manhattan Diaries, your journey into Nighttime Glamour is a testament to the allure of the city that never sleeps.

Completed Tasks: Nighttime Glamour Activities

Inspirational Quote

THE FIRST AND BEST VICTORY IS TO CONQUER ONESELF. — Plato

Action Items: Intentions and Thoughts

The Seasonal Shift

In the ever-evolving tapestry of Manhattan, each season brings with it a unique charm, an opportunity to reinvent oneself and embrace the city's transformative spirit. Just as the leaves change color in Central Park, your style should shift with the seasons, adapting to the ebb and flow of the city's energy. Join me as we explore how to navigate the seasonal shifts in Manhattan, embracing every temperature drop and warm breeze with style, grace, and, of course, a touch of that Manhattan allure.

- **Spring Fling: Blooms and Pastels**. As Manhattan awakens from its winter slumber, spring brings a burst of color and life to the city. Embrace this season with soft pastels, floral prints, and lightweight fabrics that mirror the blossoms in Central Park. Don't forget your umbrella; spring showers are an essential part of the Manhattan spring experience.

- **Sizzling Summers: Urban Heatwaves**. When summer arrives, Manhattan transforms into a concrete jungle with a tropical twist. Beat the heat with breezy sundresses, stylish sunglasses, and wide-brimmed hats. The city's parks, rooftop bars, and open-air events become your playground as you make the most of the summer sun.

- **Autumn Elegance: Falling for Fashion**. As the leaves change color, Manhattan's fashion scene takes center stage. Invest in tailored coats, cozy scarves, and ankle boots to stay both stylish and warm. Central Park's fall foliage provides the perfect backdrop for your seasonal photoshoots.

- **Winter Wonderland: Frosty Glamour**. Manhattan winters may be chilly, but they offer a chance to showcase your flair for cold-weather fashion. Bundle up in luxurious coats, oversized scarves, and chic boots. The city's holiday markets and ice skating rinks create a festive atmosphere that's perfect for holiday-inspired looks.

- **Holiday Splendor: Festive Fashion**. The holiday season in Manhattan is nothing short of magical. Embrace the spirit of celebration with glamorous cocktail dresses, sparkling accessories, and statement coats. From the iconic Rockefeller Center Christmas tree to the elaborately decorated storefronts on Fifth Avenue, let the city's festive ambiance inspire your holiday wardrobe.
- **Spring Awakening: Floral Delights**. As the city comes alive in spring, channel the energy of renewal into your style. Incorporate floral patterns, light trench coats, and playful accessories into your wardrobe. Explore Manhattan's botanical gardens and outdoor events to fully immerse yourself in the season's charm.
- **Summer Escapes: Vacation Vibes**. When the summer heat peaks, consider a stylish getaway. Pack your favorite swimsuits, airy cover-ups, and beachy accessories for a weekend escape to the Hamptons or a day trip to Coney Island. Manhattan's proximity to beach destinations offers the perfect excuse to showcase your summer fashion.

Navigating Manhattan's seasonal shifts is not just about following fashion trends; it's about embracing the unique character of each season and infusing it into your personal style. As you stroll through the city's changing landscapes, from snow-covered streets to vibrant spring blooms, let your wardrobe reflect the beauty of the ever-shifting Manhattan mosaic. In this city of constant transformation, your ability to adapt and stay stylish year-round is the ultimate testament to your Manhattan allure. So, let the seasons be your guide as you embark on this sartorial journey through the heart of Manhattan.

Completed Tasks: Seasonal Shift Activities

Inspirational Quote

LIGHT TOMORROW WITH TODAY! — Elizabeth Barrett Browning

Action Items: Intentions and Thoughts

Action Items: Intentions and Thoughts

Cocktail Hour Cleanup: Graceful and Swift Makeup Removal for the City Gal on the Go

Manhattan, a city that's as alive at the break of dawn as it is under the starry canopy. Amidst the thrumming of its vivacious heartbeat, tales of electrifying nights and hasty retreats rise like steam from its bustling streets. Navigating this wonderland, it isn't merely about making a statement; it's about transitioning with grace, from the boardroom to the ballroom, without missing a beat.

Visualize: It's the stroke of midnight. You're dashing from an opulent penthouse party on the Upper East Side to a clandestine rendezvous downtown. Every gaze locks onto you, not for the glamorous remnants of the evening, but for the pristine grace with which you've transitioned. That darling, is the Manhattan Midnight Mirage, a swift transformation that captures the essence of spontaneity and finesse.

In this invigorating chapter of The Manhattan Diaries, we delve into the discreet dance of the Cocktail Hour Cleanup. From the gentle caress of a cleansing balm to the swift swipe of a micellar-soaked cotton pad, you'll unearth the secrets to maintaining your ethereal glow, even as the night wears on.

But it's not merely about the surface, is it? It's about aligning with Manhattan's transient spirit. It's about oscillating between moments, venues, and emotions. It's about keeping pace with the city that never sleeps while ensuring that your makeup doesn't either, until you decide it's time.

So, accompany me as we meander through the luminous pathways of the city, experiencing its rhythm, its surprises, and its transitions. Understand the art of a shift that doesn't just adapt you but aligns with the city's multifaceted persona. Because, sweetheart, in Manhattan, every moment is a new scene, a fresh slate. Gird yourself, for the night is still young, and Manhattan beckons with its myriad tales. Dive into The Manhattan Diaries—where your elegance at every hour mirrors the city's timeless allure.

The Swift Makeup Removal Routine

In Manhattan's non-stop glamour, a quick and effective makeup removal routine is essential. After a dazzling night out, seamlessly transition to the comfort of home with the Swift Makeup Removal Routine. This routine is your secret to wiping the slate clean, ensuring you're ready to face another day with a fresh glow. Let's dive into the steps that keep your skin radiant, making quick transitions as effortless as the city itself.

- **Gentle Beginnings: the Night's End**. As the night winds down, it's time to prepare for your beauty transformation. Start by gently removing any false lashes, wiping away the magic of the night with a makeup remover designed for sensitive skin. This step sets the tone for a graceful transition.
- **Cleansing Balm Magic: Embrace the Meltdown**. The heart of your swift routine lies in a cleansing balm, a true magician's secret. As you massage this luxurious balm onto your skin, feel the day's stresses melt away, leaving only the softness of your natural beauty behind. It's like a moment of serenity amidst the city's chaos.
- **Micellar Marvel: The Art of Purity**. A micellar water-soaked cotton pad is your trusty companion. With a few gentle swipes, watch as it effortlessly lifts away any remnants of makeup and impurities, restoring your skin's natural clarity. This step is the epitome of elegance in simplicity.
- **Hydration Haven: Nourishing the Soul**. As the final touch, lavish your skin with a hydrating serum or moisturizer. This is the moment when you reclaim your skin's vitality, ensuring it's ready to embrace a new day of Manhattan adventures.

- **Tinted Skincare Bonus: Subtle Radiance**. For those mornings when you crave a touch of radiance, consider using a tinted moisturizer or BB cream. These multi-tasking wonders provide a sheer, natural-looking coverage while keeping your skin hydrated and protected from the city's elements.
- **Eye Makeup Perfection: Gentle Precision**. Pay extra attention to the eyes during your removal routine. Opt for an oil-based eye makeup remover to ensure a thorough yet gentle removal of mascara and eyeliner, leaving your delicate eye area refreshed.
- **Lip Love: Kissable Softness**. Your lips deserve a little extra care too. Use a gentle lip scrub to exfoliate any dryness, followed by a nourishing lip balm. This step guarantees your pout stays perfectly kissable, no matter where the city takes you next.
- **Refreshing Toner Touch: Clarifying Balance**. After cleansing, sweep a refreshing toner over your skin to refine pores and restore pH balance. This step not only refreshes your skin but also prepares it for optimal absorption of your hydrating products, ensuring your complexion remains radiant and even.
- **Soothing Eye Care: Restorative Elegance**. Conclude your routine with a targeted eye cream to soothe and hydrate the delicate eye area. This crucial step helps to reduce puffiness and diminish the appearance of dark circles, allowing you to wake up looking refreshed and ready for another day in the bustling city.

In the city that never sleeps, every moment is an opportunity for transformation. Embrace the swift makeup removal routine, where the elegance of your transitions mirrors the timeless allure of Manhattan. So, as the night turns into day, let your beauty journey be as graceful and enchanting as the city itself. After all, in Manhattan, even your morning routine can be a work of art.

Completed Tasks: Makeup Removal Activities

Inspirational Quote

OF ALL HUMAN ACTIVITIES, MAN'S LISTENING TO GOD IS THE SUPREME ACT OF HIS REASONING AND WILL.. — Pope Paul VI

Action Items: Intentions and Thoughts

The Art of Transition

Manhattan, a city that never stops, where the rhythm of life dances from one event to the next, where opportunities abound at every turn. In this whirlwind, it's not just about what you do but how seamlessly you do it. Imagine this: You're at a high-powered business meeting in Midtown, and suddenly, you receive an invite to an exclusive soiree downtown. You don't bat an eyelash; instead, you embody the Manhattan Magic-transitioning effortlessly from corporate chic to uptown glam, all without breaking a sweat.

- **Wardrobe Essentials: Transformative Pieces**. Invest in versatile wardrobe staples that effortlessly transition from day to night. A classic blazer can be draped over your shoulders during the day and paired with statement jewelry for evening allure. A little black dress is a timeless option that can be dressed up or down with accessories.
- **Quick Makeup Refresh: Effortless Glamour**. Carry a compact makeup kit in your bag, containing essentials like a neutral eyeshadow palette, a bold lipstick, and a versatile highlighter. A few strategic touch-ups can take your look from office-appropriate to cocktail chic.
- **Hair Hacks: Instant Elegance**. Learn a few easy hairstyles that can be achieved in minutes. A sleek bun or a tousled updo can transform your look from casual to sophisticated without the need for a full salon visit.
- **Accessory Swap: Statement Pieces**. Elevate your look with carefully chosen accessories. Swap out your daytime tote for a chic clutch or sling a statement necklace around your neck. Accessories are the quickest way to add drama and personality to your ensemble.
- **Grooming Essentials: On-the-Go Beauty**. Carry a small grooming kit with essentials like a nail file, blotting papers, and a

portable perfume. These quick fixes can freshen up your appearance and keep you feeling confident throughout the day and night.

- **Timing is Key: Pacing Yourself**. Master the art of time management. Keep an eye on the clock and plan your transitions accordingly. Arrive at events fashionably late, but not too late, to make a memorable entrance without rushing.
- **Confidence and Poise: The Ultimate Accessory**. No transition is complete without confidence. Believe in your ability to conquer the city's challenges and revel in its opportunities. A poised demeanor and a welcoming smile can make you the life of any party.
- **City-Ready Footwear: Comfort Meets Style**. Invest in comfortable yet stylish shoes that can take you from day to night. Opt for chic flats or low-heeled shoes for daytime comfort and switch to elegant heels or statement boots for evening glamour.
- **Strategic Layering: Adapt and Overcome**. Develop the knack for strategic layering, which allows for quick adjustments based on the occasion. This could involve pairing a sleek silk camisole under a business suit for the day and then shedding the blazer at night to showcase elegant evening wear. Layering gives you the flexibility to adapt your outfit without the need for a complete change, ensuring you're always event-ready.

As we venture through the ever-transforming streets of Manhattan, remember that your ability to transition seamlessly is a reflection of your adaptability and style. In this vibrant city, every moment presents a chance to reinvent yourself, and mastering the art of transition allows you to embrace the myriad experiences it has to offer. Welcome to The Manhattan Diaries, where your journey through the city's multifaceted landscape is a testament to your grace and versatility.

Completed Tasks: Art of Transition Activities

Inspirational Quote

I WILL LOVE THE LIGHT FOR IT SHOWS ME THE WAY, YET I WILL ENDURE THE DARKNESS BECAUSE IT SHOWS ME THE STARS. — Og Mandino

Action Items: Intentions and Thoughts

Midnight Mirage: Capturing Spontaneity

In Manhattan, where life moves fast, mastering seamless transitions is an art. From corporate meetings to chic soirees, the true Manhattanite navigates these shifts with elegance and style. Picture this: from a swanky Upper East Side party, you seamlessly glide to a downtown rendezvous, leaving a trail of admiration for your effortless grace. This is the Manhattan Midnight Mirage—spontaneity and finesse in perfect harmony.

- **Discreet Elegance: Cleansing Balm and Micellar Magic**. Discover the secrets of a swift yet effective makeup removal routine. Begin with a gentle cleansing balm that melts away the day's makeup, followed by a micellar-soaked cotton pad to cleanse and refresh your skin, leaving it ready for the next chapter of your evening.
- **Portable Beauty Arsenal: Compact Essentials**. Equip yourself with a portable beauty arsenal that includes mini-sized makeup essentials such as lipstick, mascara, and a multi-purpose palette. These compact companions ensure that you're always prepared.
- **Transition-Friendly Wardrobe: Versatile Fashion Choices**. Choose outfits that seamlessly transition from day to night. Opt for versatile pieces like a tailored blazer that pairs perfectly with office attire and can effortlessly elevate your evening ensemble.
- **Bold Statement Accessories: A Dash of Glamour**. Add a touch of drama to your look with bold accessories. A statement necklace, sparkling earrings, or a stylish clutch can instantly transform your appearance and make a striking impression.
- **Dual-Purpose Skincare: Refresh and Hydrate**. Carry a travel-sized facial mist or hydrating spray to rejuvenate your skin during transitions. A quick spritz can instantly refresh your complexion, leaving it dewy and revitalized.

- **Timeless Fragrance: Signature Scent**. Select a signature fragrance that transcends day and night. A timeless scent can create a consistent olfactory presence, making your transitions memorable and leaving a lasting impression.
- **Confidence and Poise: Inner Radiance**. The most powerful accessory is your self-confidence. Embrace every transition with poise, knowing that you carry the spirit of Manhattan within you. Your inner radiance will shine through, enhancing your overall allure.
- **Moment-Maximizing Mindset: Embrace the Unexpected**. In the city that never sleeps, transitions often lead to unexpected adventures. Maintain an open mindset, and embrace the surprises and spontaneity that Manhattan has to offer. These unexpected moments can become cherished memories.
- **Strategic Footwear: From Day to Night**. Select shoes that provide both comfort and style, allowing you to move seamlessly from daytime engagements to evening escapades. Consider versatile footwear like sleek ankle boots or convertible heels, which can adapt to any setting or style requirement, ensuring you're always step-perfect in your Manhattan journey.

In the labyrinthine streets of Manhattan, transitions are more than just moments—they're opportunities for reinvention, for embracing spontaneity, and for making your mark on the city that never sleeps. Join me as we navigate through the luminous pathways of Manhattan, capturing its transient spirit and turning every transition into a masterpiece. For in this city, every glance, every step, and every transformation is a story waiting to be told. Welcome to The Manhattan Diaries—where your elegance at every hour mirrors the city's timeless allure.

Completed Tasks: Capturing Spontaneity Activities

Inspirational Quote

WHOEVER IS HAPPY WILL MAKE OTHERS HAPPY TOO. — Anne Frank

Action Items: Intentions and Thoughts

Embracing Manhattan's Transient Spirit

In the heart of Manhattan, life moves with the speed and dazzle of Times Square. Thriving here means mastering the art of seamless transitions, from the high-energy office day to chic evening gatherings in SoHo. It's in these transformations that we capture the true essence of Manhattan—dynamic, multifaceted, and captivating. In this chapter of The Manhattan Diaries, we explore how to embrace the city's transient spirit, turning every change into an opportunity to showcase your style and grace.

- **Navigating the Dynamic Streets**. Manhattan's streets are like a symphony of change, from the iconic neighborhoods like Harlem to the Financial District. Understand that each district has its unique character, and your style should harmonize with the tempo of the moment.
- **Wardrobe Wizardry**. Embrace the power of versatile fashion choices. Layering, accessorizing, and mixing and matching pieces can effortlessly take you from day to night, ensuring you're prepared for any twist your Manhattan adventure may take.
- **Beauty on the Move**. Keep a beauty kit in your bag for quick touch-ups. A bold lip color or smoky eyeshadow can transform your look from office chic to evening elegance in seconds.
- **Transitions as Opportunities**. In Manhattan, transitions aren't just moments; they are opportunities. Be open to serendipity, as these fleeting moments can lead to unexpected connections, experiences, and memories.
- **Leveraging Technology**. Manhattan's rapid pace demands staying connected and informed. Utilize apps and digital platforms that provide real-time updates on events, transportation, and dining

options. From hailing a ride to discovering hidden gems, technology can be your ally in navigating the city's transitions seamlessly.

- **Networking with Purpose**. Embrace Manhattan's transient spirit as an opportunity to expand your network. Attend industry events, join meetups, and engage in social activities that align with your interests. The city's ever-changing landscape offers a wealth of connections waiting to be made, which can open doors to new opportunities and collaborations.
- **Cultural Adaptation**. Embracing Manhattan's transient nature also means immersing yourself in its diverse cultures. Try cuisine from different corners of the world, attend cultural festivals, and explore neighborhoods that showcase the city's rich tapestry. This not only broadens your horizons but also allows you to appreciate the dynamic blend of traditions that make Manhattan unique.
- **Self-Discovery**. The constant transitions in Manhattan provide an opportunity for personal growth and self-discovery. Use each shift as a chance to reflect on your goals, aspirations, and desires. Whether it's a change in career, lifestyle, or perspective, Manhattan's transient spirit encourages you to evolve and adapt, ultimately leading to a more profound understanding of yourself and the city you call home.

Embracing Manhattan's transient spirit is about more than just staying on the move; it's a celebration of the city's ever-evolving energy. It's an acknowledgment that, in this metropolis, change is the only constant, and your ability to adapt and thrive is a testament to your true Manhattan allure. So, step confidently through every transition, and remember, the city is your stage, and you're the star. In The Manhattan Diaries, we revel in these moments, capturing the essence of a city that never sleeps and a spirit that never wanes.

Completed Tasks: City's Transient Spirit Activities

Inspirational Quote

BE FAITHFUL TO THAT WHICH EXISTS WITHIN YOURSELF. — Andre Gide

Action Items: Intentions and Thoughts

Action Items: Intentions and Thoughts

City Roundup: The Quintessential Guide to Manhattan's Makeup Marvels

Ladies and gentlemen, in the dazzling whirlwind that is Manhattan, we've traversed the labyrinthine streets, attended exclusive soirees, and witnessed the transformative power of makeup and style. As we bid adieu to this captivating journey through "City-Slick Glamour: Manhattan's Makeup Guide to Mesmerize," we've unraveled the inner self, discovering the myriad facets that make us unique in the city that never sleeps.

From the iconic skyline to the hidden gems in each neighborhood, Manhattan's mystique has entwined with our own. We've learned that makeup isn't just about aesthetics; it's a tool to express our desires, aspirations, and the stories we want to tell.

Throughout this enchanting book, we've danced through the streets in the dewy dawn, shimmered under the sun-kissed sky, and blushed with the warmth of rosy cheeks. We've embraced the drama of Broadway, the power moves of Wall Street, and the transitions that define Manhattan's transient spirit.

We've shared secrets of graceful makeup removal, swift transformations, and the art of embracing the city's ever-changing pulse. In every step of this mesmerizing journey, we've uncovered not only the beauty of Manhattan but the beauty within ourselves.

So, as you close this book and return to the bustling streets of Manhattan, remember that you carry the allure, the glamour, and the mystique of this remarkable city with you. The Manhattan mystique isn't just in the skyline; it's in your stride, your confidence, and your unique style. Let it guide you as you continue your own Manhattan diaries, for this city has a story to tell, and you're an essential part of its narrative.

Until we meet again in the dazzling heart of Manhattan, keep mesmerizing the world with your inner self, your style, and your indomitable spirit. As The Manhattan Diaries would say, "In Manhattan, the magic never fades; it simply takes on new forms." Embrace those forms, embrace yourself, and let the mystique of Manhattan shine through you.

City-Slick Glamour Recap Checklist

The Manhattan Diaries program series recap checklist—completes step four of your 21 step journey. Think of this program as a time release supplement that does its magic over the course of 21 steps, days, or weeks—you set your schedule. By committing to one chapter each morning—or one book each day or week; in 21 short days or weeks you will be able to change your life into a new You. In this book, we covered:

1. Bright Lights, Big City, Bold Brows: Perfecting the Frame of Your Face

In this chapter of City-Slick Glamour, we dive into Manhattan's brow scene, the ultimate accessory for any city sophisticate. From the artsy streets of Greenwich Village to the polished avenues of Madison Avenue, we explore how brows frame the distinct personalities of New Yorkers. This isn't just about beauty—it's about capturing the essence of Manhattan, where each perfectly sculpted arch reflects the city's vibrant spirit. Join us as we uncover the artistry behind the city's most iconic brows, making every glance as captivating as the skyline itself.

2. Metropolitan Mattes: The Secrets Behind an Oil-Free, Photo Finish Complexion

In this chapter of City-Slick Glamour, we explore the secrets behind the Manhattan Glow—a flawless, matte complexion that's a must in the city's glamorous hustle. From the refined skincare rituals of the Upper East Side to the innovative beauty hacks of downtown trendsetters, we reveal how to achieve that perfect, oil-free finish. Here, skincare is more than a routine—it's a crucial part of your daily armor in the city that always shines. Get ready to master the art of being camera-ready with the sophistication and elegance that New York demands.

3. Rooftop Rendezvous Reds: Lip Shades for Every Occasion from Day to Night

In this chapter of City-Slick Glamour, we explore the iconic red lipsticks that define every Manhattan moment—from brunch berries to bold scarlets. Each shade is more than just color; it's a statement of confidence and allure, reflecting the city's dynamic spirit. We'll guide you through choosing the perfect red for every occasion, from daytime affairs to evening soirees, showing how a powerful pout can turn heads and capture hearts in the city that never sleeps. Join us as we celebrate the art of the red lip, a symbol of Manhattan's timeless glamour.

4. Central Park Chic: Natural Looks that Dazzle in the Daylight

In this chapter of City-Slick Glamour, we embrace the effortless elegance of Central Park Chic. Amidst the backdrop of Manhattan's skyscrapers and the natural beauty of Central Park, we explore how to achieve a radiant, natural glow. This isn't just about simple makeup; it's about harmonizing with the city's serene spirit and enhancing your natural beauty. We'll guide you through creating subtle, sunlit looks that reflect the authentic charm and vibrant energy of Manhattan, making every step through the park a showcase of understated glamour. Join us as we celebrate the art of the natural look in the heart of the city.

5. Broadway's Blushing Beauties: Achieving Cheeks that Pop and Highlight

In this chapter of City-Slick Glamour, we illuminate the art of Broadway's Blushing Beauties, exploring how to perfect cheeks that capture the spotlight. Here, we dive into techniques for applying blush and highlighter to embody the drama and elegance of Broadway. From the soft glow of a romantic lead to the bold contours of a diva, learn how each sweep of the brush enhances your narrative, mirroring the dynamic flair of Manhattan's Theater District. Step into the spotlight, darling—your radiant performance awaits.

6. The Wall Street Wing: Eyeliners that Mean Business

In this chapter of City-Slick Glamour, we focus on the Wall Street Wing—eyeliner that commands authority and signals sharp acumen. Delve into the techniques for crafting the perfect winged eyeliner that mirrors the ambition and intensity of Manhattan's financial hub. From subtle enhancements to bold declarations, learn how your eyeliner can embody your professional prowess and make every glance as impactful as your business moves. Here, your makeup is an extension of your professional persona, symbolizing power and precision on Wall Street.

7. Skyline Shadows: Eyeshadow Palettes that Mirror Manhattan's Horizon

In this chapter of City-Slick Glamour, we explore Skyline Shadows, eyeshadow palettes inspired by Manhattan's skyline. Each palette captures the city from dawn to midnight, allowing you to wear its essence on your eyelids. Here, eyeshadow is more than beauty—it's a narrative of New York, reflecting its iconic hues and moments. Dive into selecting shades that echo the city's spirit, transforming every look into a vibrant expression of Manhattan life.

8. Fifth Avenue Flutter: Lashes that Speak Volumes

In this chapter of City-Slick Glamour, we explore the enchanting Fifth Avenue Flutter, where lashes become a powerful expression of Manhattan's grandeur and mystique. Here, lashes aren't just an accessory; they narrate tales of ambition and elegance, from quiet brunches to opulent galas. We'll guide you through selecting lashes that not only enhance your look but also embody the vibrant spirit of the city. Discover how every flutter can captivate and tell stories, making each gaze a memorable part of Manhattan's lively narrative. Ready to make every blink count? Let's dive in and let your lashes do the talking.

9. The Greenwich Glow: Highlighters and Bronzers for that Gilded Finish

In this chapter of City-Slick Glamour, we delve into the Greenwich Glow, exploring how highlighters and bronzers can capture the essence of Manhattan's golden hours. From the morning's sunlit radiance to the evening's mysterious allure, we show how to embody the city's opulence with every stroke of makeup. Here, your glow tells stories of jazz bars, art-filled alleys, and historic townhouses. Learn to master a gilded finish that reflects the city's vibrant life, making your makeup a tribute to the timeless tales of Manhattan.

10. Cocktail Hour Cleanup: Graceful and Swift Makeup Removal for the City Gal on the Go

In this chapter of City-Slick Glamour, we delve into the Cocktail Hour Cleanup, teaching you quick and elegant makeup removal techniques for the bustling Manhattanite. Learn to transition flawlessly between the city's high-energy events with essentials like micellar water and cleansing balms. This guide isn't just about makeup removal; it's about keeping pace with

Manhattan's fast-paced lifestyle, ensuring you're always prepared for the next adventure. Embrace these swift, seamless methods to maintain your polish through the city's endless nights.

Where Do We Go From Here?

Darlings, as we conclude our glamorous journey through the world of "City-Slick Glamour: Manhattan's Makeup Guide to Mesmerize," we find ourselves standing at a crossroads in this dazzling city, wondering, "Where Do We Go from Here?"

Throughout these pages, we've unveiled the secrets to creating an allure that's as iconic as the Manhattan skyline itself. From the twinkling dewy dawn look to the sultry nighttime shimmer, we've embraced every facet of Manhattan's mystique. We've learned that makeup is not just a mask; it's an expression, a statement of our inner selves.

But the magic doesn't end with the final page of this book. No, my dears, it's merely the beginning. Manhattan is a city of reinvention, where change is not only embraced but celebrated. As we navigate the intricate streets and charming neighborhoods, let's carry the lessons of this journey with us.

Where do we go from here? We go forward with confidence, grace, and the knowledge that the beauty we seek is already within us. Manhattan may dazzle with its lights, but it's you who shines the brightest. Whether you're strolling through Central Park, closing deals on Wall Street, or sipping cocktails at a rooftop bar, let your inner allure radiate.

So, embrace the city's ever-changing pulse, seize the opportunities that lie ahead, and continue writing your own Manhattan diaries. Remember, it's not about where you've been; it's about where you're headed. And in the city that never sleeps, the possibilities are as limitless as your dreams.

As we part ways, take a piece of Manhattan's mystique with you, for it's an everlasting part of your story. Keep mesmerizing the world with your inner self, your style, and your indomitable spirit. The Manhattan allure never fades;

it merely evolves. Embrace that evolution, embrace yourself, and let the city's mystique guide you to new heights.

Until we meet again under the shimmering lights of Manhattan, my darlings, remember that the journey is just as enchanting as the destination. So, go forth and continue to mesmerize the world, one captivating chapter at a time.

Completed Tasks: Recap Activities

Inspirational Quote

IT'S A MOMENT THAT I'M AFTER, A FLEETING MOMENT, BUT NOT A FROZEN MOMENT. — Andrew Wyeth

Action Items: Intentions and Thoughts

Action Items: Intentions and Thoughts

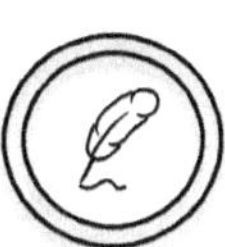

Journal Pages: Pen Your Tales

Journal Pages: Pen Your Tales

Journal Pages: Pen Your Tales

Journal Pages: Pen Your Tales

Journal Pages: Pen Your Tales

Journal Pages: Pen Your Tales

Journal Pages: Pen Your Tales

www.ingramcontent.com/pod-product-compliance
Lightning Source LLC
Chambersburg PA
CBHW021622120626
46545CB00001B/346